Murmurs in the Mountains

Smoky Mountain Secrets Saga, Book 3

Jeanne Hardt

Copyright Jeanne Hardt, 2017
Cover design by Rae Monet, Inc.
Edited by Cindy Brannam
Book formatting by Jesse Gordon

All rights reserved. No part of this publication may be reproduced, distributed, or transmitted in any form or by any means, including photocopying, recording, or other electronic or mechanical methods, without the prior written permission of the publisher, except in the case of brief quotations embodied in reviews and certain other noncommercial uses permitted by copyright law.

This book is a work of fiction. Names, characters, places, and events are the product of the author's imagination or are used fictitiously. Any likeness to actual events or persons, living or dead, is entirely coincidental. References to real places and people are intended solely for the purpose of providing a sense of authenticity.

Chapter 1

Lily's heart rested in her throat. Another change loomed ahead, and her nerves had her nearly trembling in the carriage seat. She should be used to unfamiliarity, yet her last experience had ended so badly that she feared nothing good would come to her life again.

She shut her eyes and made an effort to slow her breathing.

I can do anythin' I set my mind to.

Memories of Mrs. Gottlieb's warmness and Archibald Jones' perfect smoke rings brought a smile to her face. Not to mention, the kindness of Mr. and Mrs. Waters. She doubted they would've sent her somewhere wretched, so she shouldn't be so uneasy.

Every night, since she'd left St. Louis, she prayed the home she was going to would be loving. Mr. Jacobson *had* to be decent. Any man who donated money to a charitable cause like Water's Rest must be kind. And *good*. Hopefully, his children wouldn't be spoiled and callous.

She'd experienced enough meanness to last a lifetime.

The trip from Chattanooga had been even more impersonal than when she'd traveled to St. Louis with David. She'd paid for a seat on a stagecoach and had no interaction with the driver. They'd stopped along the way at hotels and diners, but he'd done little more than dip his head at her. Maybe he sensed she didn't want to talk.

Passengers came and went. Every now and then, Lily had made light conversation with them, but nothing more.

She'd kept essentially to herself on the steamboat as well. Though Francine Waters had assured her there were no prostitutes on that particular boat, men had sometimes looked at Lily as if they'd been told otherwise. Because of the hunger in their roaming eyes, she chose to stay in her room for the most part and had only ventured out for meals.

Now, just an hour away from her new home, she was tempted to jump from the carriage and flee in the opposite direction, back toward the cove and her son.

She opened her eyes and peered out the window. Her beloved mountains surrounded them. Their smoky haze hovered low—both beautiful and ominous.

After their last stop, only one other passenger remained. A man dressed in a well-tailored suit. She'd learned that he, too, was traveling to Asheville, but hadn't said much else. He'd spent most of the journey with his nose in a book, which suited her fine.

Her thoughts drifted, and her stomach rumbled. Without thinking, she let out a low groan.

The man cleared his throat. "Are you all right, Miss?"

She nodded and politely smiled. "I'm fine."

"Forgive me for saying this, but you look a bit peaked."

She touched a hand to her face. "Reckon I'm a mite hungry. That's all."

"Perhaps you should've exited the carriage in Waynesville and eaten with the driver and me." He tipped his head to one side and pushed out a smile. "The food at the hotel restaurant was exceptional."

Her throat closed up, and her heart thumped hard. "You're probably right," she choked out, then shifted her eyes to her lap, praying he wouldn't say anything else.

To her relief, he returned to his book.

Yes, she'd been hungry when they'd stopped in Waynesville, but she couldn't make herself budge from the seat. The chance of seeing Caleb was slim-to-none, but simply knowing he could be somewhere close had frozen her in place.

Her heart slowly steadied to a gentler pace. She withdrew Violet's letter from her pocket and clutched it tightly in her fist. Since she'd memorized every word, there was no need to read it.

David had brought the letter to her at Water's Rest the day before she'd left, along with her winter coat. To her good fortune, Evie had recovered the coat from a heap of items Aunt Helen had discarded. The weather had turned cold, and Lily appreciated the extra warmth.

Not only had she been happy to see David a final time, she'd learned Uncle Stuart had a heart after all. He'd kept the letter from Violet private. Her sister's correspondence had arrived in Lily's hand unopened, and Aunt Helen had obviously been none-the-wiser.

The letter revealed what Lily had assumed would eventually happen. Though it wasn't easy to imagine her sister married, it comforted Lily knowing Gideon was a good man.

She wished she'd been there to witness their vows. It seemed her prayers for Violet's happiness had been answered. Yet selfishly, Lily worried about Noah. With Violet gone from the cabin, it would be up to their ma to tend him. Something she'd never proven she could do. At least not as far as Lily had seen, before her forced departure.

Lily hugged the letter to her chest and sighed. Violet wanted her own baby and could very well have it before the end of next year. If she was as fertile as Lily, it would take no time at all. And once she had a child of her own, she feared Violet might forget Noah entirely.

No. Lily quickly dismissed the horrid thought. Violet was too good of a person to completely disregard him.

"Someone special?" The man gestured to the letter and set his book aside.

Lily met his gaze. "My sister. She just got married."

"That's wonderful. Marriage is a blessed thing."

She wished he'd kept reading. "Are *you* married?"

"Yes. My wife's in Asheville." He sat taller. "And what about you? Is there someone waiting to greet you upon your arrival?"

She gave a single nod. "My employer. I was hired to help a man with his four children."

"Oh. A widower?"

"No." She rapidly shook her head. "His wife had an accident and was crippled. I'll be helpin' her, too."

"I see. That's quite admirable." He rubbed his thick beard. "By any chance, is your employer Arthur Jacobson?"

Lily straightened her posture. "Yes. You know him?"

"Most everyone in Asheville is familiar with him. He manages the general store. A place people in the city frequent." He grinned, but immediately sobered. "Such a shame about his wife, but it's wonderful that you'll be assisting her."

Lily wanted to pry more information from him regarding the Jacobsons, but decided it wouldn't be proper. "They're helpin' *me*, too." She twisted her fingers into knots, wishing she'd not blurted it out.

"Oh." His brows drew together. "Did you lose your man in the war?"

His question came out of nowhere. Then again, he probably assumed the only kind of help a woman who traveled alone might need, would have something to do with a man—or lack thereof. "No. I don't *have* a man."

"A lovely woman like you? I'm surprised." He let out a small chuckle. "Forgive me. I shouldn't delve into your private affairs." With an awkward smile, he looked away, then pointed out the window. "It's a shame not all the burned buildings have been restored. I imagine it'll take some time. The war left its ugly scars everywhere. Fortunately, Asheville itself was undamaged. Physically, that is. Many residents were left poverty stricken."

Lily understood being poor and the frustrations and heartache it created. She craned her neck to see where he'd indicated. Remnants of a partially charred barn remained. "It's so sad . . ."

"Is this your first time in North Carolina?"

"Yes." She moistened her lips and swallowed hard. "I lived in St. Louis for a short time. The folks I was with acted as if the war never happened. They carried on with fancy parties an' such. It was like bein' in a different world altogether."

"You sound as if you didn't care to live there. I'd think it would be finer than having to tend someone else's children."

"No." She looked straight at him. "The place I stayed wasn't real. I'm glad to be far from it." She shut her eyes and leaned back in the seat. The man didn't press her further, no doubt sensing her need for quiet.

Her life would be utterly different if the war had ended before Ableman had arrived. She and Caleb could have openly been together, and he wouldn't have left the cove.

Revisiting all those horrid memories did no good at all. She'd torment herself forever if she constantly dwelled on what could've been.

The carriage jolted to a stop, as did her heart.

When the door opened, the man got up and stepped out. He extended a hand to help her, and since her knees were shaking, she took it. "Thank you."

"Be sure to eat something soon. You'll be no help to the Jacobsons if you faint from hunger." He kept a tight grasp on her arm until her feet were firmly planted.

Once he released her, she took a step back. "Thank you, again. You've been kind."

"Joshua?" A pretty blonde woman strode to his side. "Have you replaced me already?" She said the words with a laugh in her voice, then stood on her tiptoes and kissed his cheek.

He grabbed onto her and spun her around. "I've missed you!"

Lily couldn't help but smile. The love they held for each other shone from their eyes.

He slowly set her down again, then nodded at Lily. "Best of luck to you." Without another word or a response from her, he hastened with his wife to where the driver was unloading his belongings.

Lily looked around, hoping to be approached by someone searching for her, but no one else was about. She retrieved her knapsack from the driver, as well as a small bag Mrs. Waters had given her. It held the blue dress Lily had worn the day she'd been sent away from Aunt Helen's.

Lily no longer wore crinolines or fancy earrings, and once again, she kept her hair twisted in a single long braid down her back. She felt more like herself, but was determined to continue speaking as Mrs. Gottlieb had instructed. After all, if she wanted folks to take her seriously, she needed to prove her intelligence. She could pass on proper English to the Jacobson's children—if they hadn't already been taught to use it.

The carriage drove away, and Lily simply shrugged, standing in the center of the dusty road.

What now?

Out of nowhere, a sense of peace flooded over her. Though she was in the middle of an unfamiliar place, her beloved mountains could still be seen, framing her surroundings like a picture.

The Smokies were a part of her that truly felt like home. Somehow, she'd make this work.

She spotted Joshua and his wife a short distance away. He pointed at something behind Lily, so she spun around to see what it was.

Of course.

Stanley's General Store.

Who Stanley was, Lily wasn't sure, but certainly Joshua wouldn't point her in the wrong direction. Besides, how many general stores could there be in Asheville?

She bolstered her courage and forced her feet to move, then crossed the road and headed up the steps to the entrance.

The white wood building stood two stories tall. It looked as if it had been freshly painted and well-kept.

She went inside and gasped. Never before had she seen so much merchandise in one place. If the folks here were poverty stricken, then who would buy it all? Someone had to be able to afford all this. Maybe Joshua was mistaken. Either that, or perhaps Mr. Jacobson allowed his customers to barter or use credit. If that were true, the man was definitely generous.

She passed barrels filled with apples and potatoes. Shelves lined the wall stocked with assorted canned goods—pickled eggs, dills, honey, and many types of fruit in labeled jars. Her mouth watered and her stomach growled.

"May I help you?"

She whipped her head around and faced a tall, thin man, with wire-rimmed glasses. "Yes, sir. I'm lookin' for Mr. Jacobson."

He smiled. "Actually, you're looking *at* him."

His pleasant expression warmed her all the way to her bones. "Oh. Well, I'm Lily. Lily Larsen . . . You know . . . from St. Louis." Her nerves had gotten the best of her, and she stammered out her words. Since she had no idea what Mr. and Mrs. Waters had told him about her, he could very well think she'd been a prostitute. That notion didn't set well, but she doubted she'd ever tell him the real reason she'd been sent to Water's Rest.

His eyes widened. "Oh, dear." He jerked a watch from his pocket and flipped it open. "I was counting my inventory and lost track of time. I'd intended to meet you when the stage arrived. Please, forgive me."

"There's nothin' to forgive. You're a busy man." She glanced around the store and didn't see a single patron. "That is . . . I'm sure there's plenty to do here. Especially if you have to count everythin'." The interior of the store was twice the size of her cabin in the cove.

"Yes, there's much to tabulate. But there's far more that needs tending at my home."

She returned his generous smile. He definitely didn't sound like he was from the south. Lily wanted to know more about him, yet now wasn't the time to ask. If she acted overly curious or nosy, he might think she was rude.

He tucked the timepiece back into his pocket. "I'll close up shop and take you to the house. Arabelle is looking forward to meeting you." He scurried down the aisle, locked the door, then flipped the sign in the window to *closed*.

"That's a lovely name. I assume Arabelle is your wife?"

"Yes. And my children are Winnifred, Genevieve, Opal, and Levi. But, I'm getting ahead of myself. It will be best to introduce them when you can put their individual features with their names." His eyes narrowed and he searched Lily's face. "I'm glad you came. I was assured you're kind-hearted. It's important that I have someone loving to take care of my family."

With every word he spoke, her nervousness eased. "I'll do my best. I hope they like me."

He gestured to a door at the back of the building and moved toward it. "My children have struggled since Arabelle's accident. She used to play with them. Now, she has many limitations."

Lily followed him outside. They silently walked a short distance down the road to a livery. She waited beside the large open door while he retrieved his horse and buggy.

He halted right next to her and started to get out to help her, but she waved him down. "I can manage." She carefully lifted her skirt, stepped up onto the floorboard, and sat.

He smiled and snapped the reins. "It's not far." His shoulders slumped, and he stared vacantly forward. "When we first arrived, we lived in the apartment above the store. There are stairs on the side of the building that lead up to it. *Steep* stairs. Arabelle always fretted over the children managing them. Then, one day, while ascending, she turned sharply to chastise the girls for arguing. She lost her footing and stumbled sideways against the handrail. It had been poorly constructed and gave way. She fell to the ground. Fortunately, she didn't strike her head, but the impact broke her back and paralyzed her from the waist down."

The pain in his voice broke Lily's heart. "I'm so sorry."

His head slowly bobbed. "I found a small house just outside the city that suits us."

He fell silent, and Lily gave him his peace. Heart aching, she grasped the seat with both hands. Soon, she'd meet her new family, yet she yearned for the one she'd left behind in the cove.

Chapter 2

Mr. Jacobson brought the buggy to a stop in front of a white wood house. It looked as if it had been freshly painted in the same manner as the store. A picket fence lined the small yard that surrounded it. It hadn't been afforded the expensive paint, but appeared as if it had a nice whitewash.

Lily caught sight of what appeared to be an attempt at a vegetable garden. Though many weeds had grown and overpowered it, a few pumpkins and winter squash poked through the mess.

Mr. Jacobson sighed. "You noticed our pitiful garden?"

She nodded. "Don't fret. Next year I'll have it puttin' out more vegetables than y'all can eat. But I imagine you get plenty a food from your store."

"Yes, thank goodness. If we had to rely on our own means, we'd starve. Even so, there's something rewarding about consuming food you've harvested with your own two hands. From what you said, I assume you know something about working the ground?"

She lifted her chin high. "Yes, sir. I farmed most a my life, an' I love doin' it."

He hopped to the ground and helped her from the buggy. "It seems Mr. and Mrs. Waters sent me an angel."

She folded her hands in front of herself and looked directly at him. "I'm no angel, but I'm not afraid to work hard. More than anythin', I appreciate you bringin' me here an' givin' me a chance."

He smiled—something she found he did a lot. "Everyone deserves the opportunity to better their life."

"Mine hasn't been what I expected, but I'm doin' my best to make the most of it."

"That's all any of us can do. If we lived each day being bitter about unexpected circumstances, our hearts would turn cold and we wouldn't be the joyful people God intends us to be."

"With all you've been through, don't you find it hard bein' happy?"

"At times." He solemnly nodded. "But I wake up each morning, thankful to be alive—and my family with me. Not everyone is so fortunate." He glanced at the house, then shifted his eyes toward the horse and buggy. His brows wove, and he nervously rubbed his chin. "Would you mind waiting here a few moments while I settle the horse in the barn? I'll be quick about it. I'd prefer to escort you inside rather than send you in alone."

"I don't mind waitin' at all. I'll stay glued to this spot till you return."

"Thank you." He hopped back into the buggy and drove it behind the house. Within moments, he was scurrying toward her again.

"That *was* fast," she said with a laugh. "I barely blinked."

Grinning, he pushed open a gate and led her along a stone pathway. With another pleasant smile, he spun on his heels and opened the front door.

Lily was speechless. After so many months of feeling sorry for herself, maybe she'd start to heal if she had an attitude like Mr. Jacobson's.

A small boy rushed toward them as fast as his little body allowed. He wrapped his arms around Mr. Jacobson's legs, then peered upward. His hair was so blond it was almost white and his plump cheeks made him adorable. Seeing him also brought an ache to Lily's heart.

The man grinned and picked him up. "This is Levi."

Lily's throat closed up and tears threatened. She'd not expected to have such a strong reaction to the boy.

I'm such a mess.

She took a calming breath. "Hello, Levi."

He shyly buried his face against his pa's shoulder.

The man chuckled. "Don't worry. He'll warm up to you. Oh—and speaking of *warm*—you can hang your coat there." He gestured to a hook beside the front door.

Lily gladly did so. A fire blazed in the corner of the room and proficiently heated the house. Fortunately, the time she took hanging her coat gave her a few moments to get her mind right.

"Father's home early!" The cry came from the back of the house.

Three young girls appeared dressed in frilly dresses that looked more appropriate for Sunday services. An odd thing to wear on a weekday.

Lily glanced down at her simple brown garment, feeling underdressed and plain. But she hadn't come here to make a physical impression, she'd come to help and had dressed accordingly.

The girls rushed across the room, then abruptly stopped when they eyed Lily. Though each of them had a different shade of hair, they all had similar facial features—tiny button noses, high cheekbones, and very pretty.

Lily stood silently and waited for an introduction.

The youngest of the girls stepped closer. "Are you Lily?"

"Miss *Larsen*," her pa corrected and nodded at Lily. "Opal tends to be outspoken."

Lily smiled at her. "You an' I already have sumthin' in common."

Opal giggled, all the while winding a strand of her long blond hair around her finger. "But I'm only five. You're a lot bigger than me." Another giggle. "I like the way you talk."

"She's from the south," the tallest girl said. "I can tell by her accent." She shifted away from her sister and looked straight at Lily. "I know things because I'm older than them." She pointed a thumb at her sisters. "*I'm* eleven, but Father says I act more grownup than most girls my age." She tilted her head to one side and dissected Lily with her eyes. "Where are you from?"

Her pa shifted Levi onto one hip, then put an arm over the girl's shoulder. "Winnifred. You must give me time to introduce you before you pry Miss Larsen for information."

Winnifred screwed her lips together. "Please don't call me that, Father. I told you, I want to be called *Winnie*." She returned her gaze to Lily. "Will *you* call me Winnie?"

"Of course. If that's what you prefer."

The girl beamed.

The final of the three—no doubt, Genevieve—smirked. "I'm only nine, but I'm just as smart as she is." She rolled her eyes at Winnie. "*I* think we should call her *Fred*. She runs around acting like a boy all the time, climbing trees and catching bugs. It's so unladylike." She hoisted herself primly straight, jerked her head high, and tossed her reddish hair.

Winnie butted against Genevieve with her shoulder. "You're not as smart as me, and don't *ever* call me Fred." Again, her features puckered. "Father, make her behave."

Genevieve pushed back. "*You're* the one acting poorly."

"No, I'm not."

"Yes, you are!"

The two faced each other, scowling.

"That's enough!" Mr. Jacobson stomped his foot. His harsh outburst startled Lily, but it made sense. From what he'd told her, the girls' bickering had led to his wife's accident.

He inhaled deeply and stood taller. "You're making a terrible first impression on Miss Larsen." His voice regained its calm. "Now, tell each other you're sorry."

"Sorry," they both grumbled.

Opal giggled harder, and Levi clung to his pa without making a sound.

For the first time in a very long while, Lily felt at home. The Jacobsons were a *real* family, and she already adored the children. However, she worried they might be a bit spoiled. Their attire alone showed evidence of pampering.

"Forgive them," Mr. Jacobson said. "They usually get along quite well."

"They're fine." Lily smiled at each child in turn. "Truth be told, y'all remind me of my family back home."

"Father?" Winnie moved close to him. "Is it all right if I ask her *now* where she's from?"

He smiled and nodded, and Winnie questioned Lily with her eyes.

"I'm from Cades Cove in Tennessee," Lily said. "Not too far from here. It's a beautiful place deep in the Smokies." Talking about it broadened Lily's smile.

Winnie studied her face. "Why'd you leave there?"

The long, complicated story was too harsh for any child to hear, so Lily simplified it. "I left, so I can care for y'all."

"And our mother?" Winnie's sad eyes tugged at Lily's heart. Being the eldest, Winnifred probably understood the seriousness of her ma's condition even more so than the other children.

"Yes." She smoothed a hand down Winnie's chocolate-colored hair. "But I'll likely need your help, too. I'm not familiar with anythin' here. Can I count on you to help me?"

"Me, too?" Genevieve glued herself to Lily's side.

"And me?" Little Opal joined her.

"*All* of you," Lily said. "Even Levi." She grinned at the boy, who quickly turned his head and once again buried his face against his pa's shirt.

Opal tugged on Lily's skirt. "You're lovely. Father didn't tell us *that*."

The child's remark warmed Lily's cheeks. "Thank you, that's very kind."

Mr. Jacobson set Levi down, but the boy remained at his feet. "Is your mother resting?"

"Yes," Winnie said. "She had a bad morning. The woman from church didn't come to help."

"Oh, dear." Mr. Jacobson swallowed hard. "Look after the others while I take Miss Larsen to meet your mother."

"Yes, sir." Winnie took Levi by the hand and led him off into another room. Genevieve and Opal followed.

Lily watched them go. "The children are certainly obedient."

"Yes. They're very good. *Most* of the time."

Lily had wanted to pick Levi up and hold him, but she understood the importance of giving him the time he needed to feel comfortable with her. The essence of her own son—even his unique smell—lingered in her memory. Somehow, she had to find a way to see him again.

Mr. Jacobson guided her down a short hallway and entered a bedroom. He held up a single hand and stopped Lily in the doorway. "Give me a moment."

"All right."

He pushed the door almost shut.

Lily pressed herself against the wall and patiently waited. Soft murmurs came from the room, mixed with what sounded like crying. Mr. Jacobson's voice remained calm and soothing, though Lily couldn't discern what he was saying.

The door inched open. "Come in. I'll show you what has to be done."

Mrs. Jacobson lay in the bed covered with numerous quilts. And though the room was a bit cold, it didn't seem to warrant so many blankets.

"This is Arabelle." Mr. Jacobson sat on the edge of the bed and stroked his wife's long brown hair. "Arabelle, dear, I'd like you to meet Lily Larsen."

Lily stepped closer. "I'm pleased to meet you, ma'am."

"Hello." The word came out in a weak whisper, followed by a sniffle.

Mr. Jacobson dabbed at her nose with a handkerchief. "My wife is upset because there was no one here to change her."

Another sniffle.

"You see," he went on, "we've been blessed with the service of several church ladies who take turns caring for her while I'm working. But, as Winnifred indicated, the woman didn't come. I had told them you were arriving today, so they must've assumed they were no longer needed."

"So," Lily whispered, "she needs to be changed." Lily jutted her chin, then laid a hand on the woman's arm. Since Mrs. Jacobson was paralyzed from the waist down, she wouldn't be able to control her bodily functions. No wonder she was so upset. She required care similar to that of a baby. "I'll help you. You don't hafta cry." She turned to Mr. Jacobson. "Show me where her things are, as well as a wash basin an' rags."

He stood. "You don't mind?"

"Course not. It's what I came for. Your poor wife should never hafta lay there unattended."

"So, this doesn't disturb you?"

"I've looked after all my siblin's. An' whenever my ma an' pa was sick, I took care a them, too. There's not much a anythin' that bothers me."

He shut his eyes, then slowly opened them again. "You truly are an angel." He glanced back at his wife. "Sweetheart, I'll get the water to wash you. I'll leave Lily here, so you can become better acquainted." With a quick nod, he left the room.

Lily gingerly sat on the side of the bed where he'd been. "Do you mind, ma'am?"

"You can call me Arabelle."

"It's a beautiful name. I've never heard it before." Lily pulled the blanket away from Arabelle's face, finding her as lovely as the girls. "Your daughters look just like you." She smiled, then picked up the handkerchief Mr. Jacobson had left behind and wiped away Arabelle's tears.

Lily decided to be bold. "I can't imagine what it must be like not havin' the ability to walk or do all the things you used to do. I'll try as hard as I can to make things easier for you."

"Thank you. I hope you're accustomed to a great deal of work. There's so much to be done—and my children are too young to help."

"You might be surprised. I reckon I can teach your little ones to do more around here than you realize. When I was Winnie's age, I was sowin' wheat an' skinnin' rabbits."

"Oh?" She pushed with her hands and tried to scoot up higher on her pillow, but her thin arms trembled, and she made no progress.

Lily helped her. "Yep." She readjusted the blankets. "Aren't you hot under all these?"

"No. I have difficulty staying warm. It's another issue with my paralysis. I'm either too hot or too cold."

Mr. Jacobson walked in with a pan of water. He set it on a small table, then shut the door.

Lily's compassion for his disabled wife moved her to act. She hadn't lied. The task at hand didn't disgust her, she saw it as a way to help. Tending Mrs. Jacobson took Lily beyond her own self-pity. There were many folks less fortunate than herself, and if she could make a positive difference to this sweet family, she would give it her all.

* * *

Once Lily had helped Arabelle clean herself and dress in a fresh gown, Lily left her to rest—something she claimed she needed. Truthfully, Lily found it odd that she constantly laid around in her bed clothes. She believed the woman should get up, dress in daywear, and help set the house straight.

A wheelchair sat in the corner of the room, so Arabelle had the means to get around. From what Lily understood, she had full use of her hands and arms, and apparently had a sharp mind. Lying in bed all day only weakened her muscles and wasted away her life. Her children needed her, as did her husband.

However, since Lily had arrived only hours prior, she knew it wasn't her place to point out the obvious. Maybe in time.

When Lily had first entered the house, she'd been so focused on the children that she'd taken in little of the interior. Now that Mrs. Jacobson was settled, Lily's eyes were opened to the vast amount of work needing to be done.

Dirty dishes were piled high on the kitchen counter, clothes were strewn about, and it looked as if the floor hadn't been swept in weeks. The furnishings appeared expensive, but were in such disarray that it took away from their fineness.

The Jacobsons didn't need an angel, they desperately required a maid.

"Time to get busy," Lily muttered, then spotted Mr. Jacobson heading for the kitchen.

He grabbed an apron from a peg on the wall and tied it around his waist. The sight made Lily grin, but she quickly covered it. She couldn't imagine her pa ever donning any sort of feminine garment.

Those thoughts took her straight to Caleb, but the sharp wrench in her heart forced her to dismiss the memory of him in a dress.

Levi scurried into the room and entwined himself once again around his pa's legs. He was the perfect distraction. The sweet boy eyed Lily, yet before she had a chance to even smile at him, he covered his face with his pa's pantleg.

Lily wandered into the kitchen. "Arabelle's restin'. I'm ready to do whatever you'd like me to. Want me to fix supper?"

"You can cook?" He took a step toward her. At the same time, Levi circled his leg with his arms and held on tight.

Mr. Jacobson teetered and clutched the corner of the counter. He'd nearly been toppled by the toddler.

Lily giggled and squatted down to the boy's level. "You're strong. How old are you?" She touched her finger to the tip of his nose.

He didn't utter a sound and simply blinked.

"Can you at least tell me hello?" She hoped he *could* speak. She'd not yet heard evidence of it.

Mr. Jacobson picked him up. "He just turned two. Didn't you, Levi?"

The boy gazed at his pa, but remained silent.

Mr. Jacobson lightly jostled his arm. "Say hello to Miss Larsen, Levi."

He shook his head *no*.

"My son tends to be shy." Mr. Jacobson bounced him up and down a few times. "C'mon now, say *something*. Anything you want to say."

"I hungry." Levi pointed at the stove. "Make food."

Though the child sounded demanding, hearing him speak eased Lily. She tenderly placed a hand on his head. "I'll fix sumthin' right up." She had no idea what was available to cook, but assumed there'd be an abundance of food from the store.

Finally, the child smiled at her. It warmed her all the way to her toes.

"Excellent," Mr. Jacobson said. "I'll show you where everything is, and you can help yourself to whatever you need. Then I'll attempt to clean up some of this mess. I'm sorry you have to see our house in such disorder. Arabelle was extraordinary at keeping house. But now—"

"It's fine." Lily grabbed another apron and put it on. "Where have the girls gotten off to?"

"They like to play outside, so as not to disturb their mother."

Lily thrust her chin high. There was no time like the present to be bold. "What 'bout their chores? Don't they help tidy up?"

"Not exactly. We believe children shouldn't be burdened with menial labor. At times, we've asked them to pick up their toys, but for the most part we encourage their playtime and use of their imaginations. I've always been able to provide for them, and until Arabelle's accident, our household ran smoothly."

Lily politely nodded. What she truly wanted to do was fetch the girls and get them working. For tonight, she'd let them be, but tomorrow was another day. And once their pa left for the store, they would be under her supervision. She intended to teach the children that they were an important part of this family and especially under the circumstances, they needed to do more than play.

The children dressed and spoke properly. They sounded like they'd come from somewhere in the North. Lily had thought she might need to pass on what Mrs. Gottlieb had taught her, but the lessons these folks required had been inbred in Lily. Habits she'd taken on since she'd been old enough to walk. She'd assumed everyone understood the necessity of pulling together to get things done. No matter their age. All the *properness* in the world couldn't accomplish that.

A new kind of fluttering filled Lily's belly, and she couldn't help but smile. These folks needed her more than they realized. The possibilities of making a positive change in their lives excited her.

It finally felt like her life might be headed in the right direction.

Chapter 3

Caleb's head jerked upright. He'd fallen asleep in the living room chair, exhausted from harvesting the corn, and a knock on the front door brought him out of his stupor.

Another, more persistent rap resounded.

He shook his head to cast off drowsiness, then stood and hastened to the door.

"Ma?" He looked beyond her to the near-dark sky. "What are you doin' here so late? Becca an' Avery's already in bed."

"Good. It's you I need to talk to." She nodded toward the interior. "Are you gonna let me in?"

"Course." He stepped aside.

She quickly brushed past him and continued on into the kitchen.

He shrugged and followed her. "Sumthin' wrong?" The house was utterly quiet, so he kept his voice low to make certain he didn't rouse his family. Whenever his ma wanted to talk to him alone, it was never good.

As silently as they could, they took their places at the table.

"I tried settlin' in for the night," his ma whispered, "but my mind wouldn't rest. I could tell yesterday at supper that sumthin' was botherin' Rebecca. I thought the two a you had worked out all your problems."

"We have. *Mostly.*" He leaned back in his chair and looked her in the eye. "She was ill cuz her flow came again. I wish she'd just stop frettin' 'bout havin' another baby an' be happy with what we got."

"Rebecca has one of the happiest dispositions of any soul on earth. Hmm . . . She was likely feelin' discomfort from her time. You're well aware it's not pleasant for women."

"No. It's more than that." At times Caleb wished his ma wouldn't be so blunt. "She cried last night 'bout not conceivin'."

"Are you lovin' on her like you should?"

He shut his eyes and lowered his head. "Heavens sakes, Ma. I don't like talkin' 'bout all that with you. But yes, I'm doin' what needs to be done."

"Hmm . . ." She thrummed her fingers on the table. "Maybe *you're* the problem."

"But I just told you—"

"I know. You're doin' what you should. An' we know full well Rebecca is capable of conceivin', so I reckon your seed ain't no good."

He gaped at her, then leaned across the table and lowered his voice even more. "But what 'bout Noah?"

"Who's Noah?" Her eyes pinched into slits, and she scowled. "That the name a the Larsen girl's boy?"

He let out a long breath and sat back again. "Yes. I thought I told you. I musta never mentioned his name."

"Nope. You didn't." Sighing, she gazed upward. "Noah . . ." she mumbled, then snapped her head down and stared right at him. "As I told you before—"

"*Shh.*" Caleb held up a hand and widened his eyes.

His ma bent forward. "As I said," she whispered. "I wouldn't believe a word Lucas Larsen told you. If there's a baby at all, it's likely *Mrs.* Larsen's. Lucas only wanted to hurt you by tellin' you it's yours. Mark my word."

"I hope you're right. But if you are, then why'd they send Lily away?"

His ma pulled her shoulders back and sat upright. "Maybe she *wanted* to leave. You broke the girl's heart, son. Sometimes a woman needs to distance herself from a place where she was hurt."

He slumped in his seat. "That makes me feel *so* much better." His sarcasm came through clearly.

"Well. The truth is painful. I'm afraid your past will always be hurtful, an' unfortunately, your future will likely have even more disappointments. I believe you an' Rebecca may never have a child of your own. I truly think you got infertile seed."

He shook his head and stared at the table. He didn't believe that for a minute. But then again, why *hadn't* Rebecca conceived?

His life would be far less complicated if he could convince himself that he hadn't left Lily burdened with a pregnancy. It would ease at least *some* of his guilt.

As many falsehoods as Lucas had created, Noah could be a lie, too. Yet, for some odd reason, Caleb believed everything Lucas had told him about the boy. Caleb felt deep inside himself that the child was real *and* his son. And though his ma had made it clear that he should stay far away from the Larsens, he yearned to return to the cove. Something kept tugging him in that direction.

"Caleb?" His ma waved a hand in front of his face. "Get your mind right. I can tell you're thinkin' things you shouldn't. You got your mind on Lily, don't ya?"

He held a finger to his lips and widened his eyes at the woman. "Please don't say her name here."

"Well, *you* did."

Sometimes, when they had these kind of discussions, his ma felt more like a sibling than a parent—someone to argue with rather than take advice from. "I wasn't thinkin' 'bout her, I had my mind on the boy."

"You best start tellin' your *mind* that child don't exist. Hear me?" She tapped the tip of her finger on the table. "Have I ever led you in the wrong direction?"

He stared at her, unable to say what he wanted to. If she hadn't pushed him so hard in Rebecca's direction, he'd likely be with Lily now.

With a huff, his ma waved a hand at him, then folded her arms across her chest. "I only want what's best for you. That's all."

"I know, Ma." He blinked several times, then met her gaze. "I'm tired. Reckon I need to get to bed." He jerked his head toward the window. "An' since it's dark outside, you best be stayin' here t'night. You shouldn't be walkin' to the hotel this late."

"Thank you. Is my bed made up?"

He grunted a laugh. "Course it is. But promise me when you go by Avery's room, you won't wake her."

"Well, you know I gotta give her a kiss." She stood and cocked her head. "I love that baby. I'll do my best to give her a quiet little peck."

"I appreciate it." He carefully scooted his chair back and rose to his feet, then bent sideways and stretched. "It's been a long day."

"That it has." She walked around the table and hugged him. "You're a hard worker, Caleb. I'm proud a the way you brought this farm back to life." Smiling broadly, she patted his cheek. "Now, get on to bed an' hold that wife a yours. I'll get up early an' fix y'all a good breakfast."

"Thank you. I know Becca will appreciate it, too."

With another pat to his face, she headed down the hallway.

He leaned against the wall and watched her tiptoe into Avery's room. No cry came, nor did any sounds of his daughter's babbling. Soon, his ma came out, gave him a quick glance over her shoulder, then went into her bedroom and shut the door.

They'd set it up for her the way she liked it, so it would be ready whenever she spent the night. They'd even suggested she forego her room at the hotel and move in with them, but she insisted it wouldn't be wise. She'd said firmly that every young couple required private space.

Caleb assumed his ma needed her own privacy. Not merely a bedroom in their house. She was still a lovely woman, not yet forty. If the war hadn't taken the lives of so many men, she'd likely have remarried. But decent husbands were hard to come by. Regardless, it was difficult for Caleb to picture her with anyone but his pa. On the other hand, he didn't want her to grow old alone. Maybe fate would lend a hand.

* * *

Rebecca had barely slept a wink, though she'd pretended to be sleeping when Caleb had come to bed. He'd cuddled up behind her, but she gave no reaction. She hadn't been in the mood for his affections.

She'd heard his ma arrive, and shortly thereafter bits and pieces of an intense conversation between her and Caleb.

The name, *Lily*, had come through crystal clear more than once.

From the first time Rebecca had been told of Lily Larsen, she'd felt uneasy about the girl. Something in the way Caleb had said her name, and the expression on his face when it passed his lips. Rebecca's anxiousness over Lily hadn't subsided, but she wasn't about to ask Caleb about her. If something had truly transpired between the two of them, it had happened in the past. Long before Caleb had married her. Therefore, it shouldn't matter in the least.

The past month with Caleb had been wonderful. He'd been paying extra attention to her, and they'd laughed more than they ever had. Until last night, the only thing that bothered her was not conceiving. But now, Lily Larsen had returned to the forefront of her mind and brought an additional worry.

The scent of frying bacon caused her mouth to water. Her mother-in-law never burned food, and they were sure to have a good breakfast.

Caleb appeared in the doorway of their bedroom holding Avery. "Good. You're awake. Ma's fixin' breakfast."

Rebecca sat up, then swung her legs around and planted her feet on the floor. "I can smell it." She stood and put on a robe. "She musta come over last night. Why didn't you wake me up?"

Caleb crossed to her and kissed her forehead. "I knew you was tired."

"So, why'd she come over? 'Specially so late?"

He let out an uncomfortable-sounding laugh. "She said she couldn't sleep, so she came by to visit."

"Oh." She knew there was more to it, but wouldn't press him. His nervous chuckle told her a great deal, yet if she kept worrying over every little thing, she'd be a mess.

They headed for the kitchen. The closer they got, the aroma of coffee overtook the bacon.

"Mornin', Ma." Rebecca nodded at the frying pan. "Need help with the hotcakes?"

"No. You go on an' sit down. I got this." She poured batter into the pan.

Avery's face lit up. She clapped her hands and squealed.

"She loves your hotcakes," Caleb said and sat with her on his lap.

Rebecca pushed out a smile and took her place beside them. "We all do."

Her mother-in-law glanced over her shoulder, grinning.

Had it not been for Rebecca's deep-seated fears, she'd enjoy this kind of pampering. But her heart couldn't rest.

Maybe she'd have to try a bit harder and cast her worries aside.

Chapter 4

Violet cuddled against Gideon's chest. "It's so cold. Can't we stay in bed a little longer?"

He drew his fingers through her hair. "Nope. Rooster crowed a while ago. You know we got a lot to do. Winter wheat needs to be sown, an' Ma's been harpin' 'bout pickin' apples." He hoisted himself up on one elbow and peered down at her. "I'd like nothin' more than to spend all day here with you, but my folks are countin' on us."

She stuck out her lower lip, hoping to draw on his sympathy. "Fifteen more minutes?" To further entice him, she glided her fingers over his bare skin. "Please? I'd like you to warm me up real good 'fore we get out from under these covers."

"You ain't playin' fair, Violet."

She circled his navel with her fingertip, grinning.

He trembled. "You know what that does to me."

"Yep." She giggled and yanked him to her.

After being married almost a full month, they'd gotten to know each other well. She cherished these moments alone with him. It was their private time to love on each other and share their most intimate thoughts and feelings.

Their kisses alone heated her body, and when they joined, she became lost in him. He was gentle but intense, and whenever they coupled, it became even more enjoyable. Something she didn't think possible. Love had made her deliriously happy.

She had to refrain from giggling whenever he released. His face always puckered and twisted like he'd tasted something sour, then he'd cry out and his entire body would fold down onto her. Once his breathing calmed, he'd let out a happy sigh and roll off her.

She could tell he was close. Whenever he left his seed in her, it brought the wonderful possibility of a child. She squirmed with joy. "I love you, Gideon."

He moaned and rose up high. His eyes squinted shut and his face puckered.

Here it comes.

"Bless it!" He always cried out with the same words. It tickled her, but she'd never laugh at him. Nothing brought her more happiness than knowing how much he enjoyed having her.

His body went rigid, then he flopped down like a ragdoll.

"My sweet Gideon," she whispered in his ear and tenderly caressed his back.

He lifted his head and cast a goofy grin. "Now I wanna sleep some more." With a sigh, he rolled over into his own space.

She turned on her side and again burrowed against him. "We can't. We got work to do, remember?"

"You're an evil woman." He narrowed his eyes.

"But you love me, right?"

"More than anythin'." He kissed her forehead. "We best be gettin' our tails over to the cabin. Ma's been understandin' of how late we've been—bein' newlyweds an' all—but I know she don't like breakfast gettin' cold."

Gideon flung the blankets aside and sat up. No matter how many times Violet saw his stumped leg, it still pained her. She wasn't disgusted by it in any way, but it broke her heart knowing how he'd suffered, both physically and emotionally.

He kept his crutch close to the bed and easily hoisted himself onto his lone foot.

Violet shivered and pulled the sheet over herself. "We shoulda put a bigger log on the fire last night. It's barely smolderin'."

"Get up an' get movin' an' you'll be fine." He grinned. "I hafta admit, I like lookin' at you lyin' there. You take my breath."

She sat up, still hugging the sheet to her body. "Get some clothes on Gideon Myers, or I'll yank you back down here again."

He hobbled close, bent over, and kissed her. "I'll be thinkin' 'bout that all day. I ain't never gonna get enough a you."

"Good." She placed her hands atop her belly. "Reckon we already made a baby?"

He beamed. "I hope so. You'll be the best ma ever."

"I'll sure try." She sighed and stood from the bed. "I wanna go see Noah today. Make sure he's doin' all right. Do you mind?"

"Course not. I'd go with you, but Pa needs my help." He set his clothes out on the bed, then started dressing. "Can you come back soon enough to pick apples? Ma's gettin' anxious 'bout cannin' some sauce for winter."

Violet tugged on her undergarments. "I won't be gone long. I know I'm needed here, too."

"Yep. 'Specially by me."

Their eyes locked for a brief moment. The love in the air completely warmed her.

They finished dressing, then hand-in-hand, headed the short distance to the main cabin.

The small weaner house suited Violet. She admitted, she hated housework, and it was easy straightening up her tiny place. She didn't mind exerting herself, but preferred the idea of being a ma and tending children. That was the kind of work she'd been made for.

* * *

After thanking her mother-in-law for a delicious breakfast, Violet went to the barn and readied Stardust for the short ride to her folks' cabin. Her pa had graciously given her the mare shortly after she and Gideon married, as a special wedding gift. She couldn't have asked for anything more wonderful.

She'd tried several times to get Gideon to ride the horse. At first, he'd said he wasn't ready, but his response eventually became an adamant *no*. He swore that a one-legged man had no business riding and claimed to be content going from place to place in his folks' buggy. But Violet loved to ride and wished her husband shared her fondness for it.

She took her time riding to the old cabin. With so much beauty surrounding her, it would've been sinful not to appreciate it. She loved every season in the mountains, yet fall was her favorite. More colors than a rainbow dotted the mountainside. The trees were always the prettiest right before their leaves began to drop and bare every limb.

The fall also had its own unique clean smell. The very essence of the cove soothed her. Though it had definitely changed since the war—mostly because of the loss of many loved ones—it had started to regain its peace. Folks had set aside their differences and had come together again as a loving community.

How could she ever have thought of leaving this incredible place? Poor Lily had been forced out. At least Violet could do right by her sister and make certain Noah was well.

Since she planned to visit for several hours, she put Stardust in her old stall, then headed for the cabin. Now that it was no longer her home, she lightly rapped on the door to make her presence known, then slowly pushed it open and stepped inside. "It's me, Ma."

"Good timin'." Her ma sat at the kitchen table, knife in hand. "You can help peel these apples." Two large buckets nearly overflowed with them.

Not exactly what Violet had in mind, but she couldn't tell her ma *no*. She got another paring knife from a drawer and took a seat beside her. "Horace an' Isaac pick these?"

"Yep."

The house was utterly silent. "They out helpin' Pa in the fields?"

"Mmm, hmm."

"Noah must be takin' a nap." Violet cautiously peeled each apple. She'd cut herself more than once on prior occasions.

"Nope. Noah ain't here."

Violet's stomach twisted and she gaped at the woman. "Where is he?"

Her ma's eyes lifted from her work, and she met Violet's gaze. "Don't look at me like that. I done what I had to. He started walkin' last week and gets under foot all the time. I can't be expected to get anythin' done 'round here tendin' that boy. An' your pa an' brothers hafta work the fields. They can't help with him neither."

The dryness in Violet's throat couldn't be relieved no matter how hard she swallowed. "But where'd you take him?" She laid down the knife.

"Mrs. Henderson is watchin' him. Her twins keep him entertained, an' she claims it helps her. They're enthralled with the boy."

"But the twins ain't much older than Noah. How can it help her havin' *three* little ones underfoot?"

Her ma huffed. "I don't know, an' I don't rightly care. If she's happy to do it, then so be it."

"If he's all that trouble, why don't you let me take him? I'd be glad to watch him. You *know* that."

"Course I do. An' it's the very reason I won't have you doin' it. That boy is confused enough as it is. The two a you was too close."

"How can I be too close to my nephew?" Heat coursed through Violet's veins.

"*Brother*! Get that through your skull 'fore you slip an' say the wrong thing in front of someone who matters." She jerked her head toward the buckets of apples. "Now, get to peelin' an' keep your mind on the task at hand."

Violet begrudgingly picked up the knife. She clamped her mouth shut and hissed air through her nostrils.

She'd never treat her children the way her ma treated hers. But with each apple Violet peeled, her anger lessened and eventually turned to sorrow. Her ma hadn't always been this way. Violet recalled the loving woman who'd rock her to sleep at night. But once the boys came, they'd been rocked mostly by Lily.

Their ma got even worse when the war started. She fretted all the time. And when their pa came home without an arm, the woman turned bitter. Now, they all suffered for it.

They worked in silence.

Violet sliced her way through several dozen apples. She'd calmed enough to ask about the other issue that she'd been losing sleep over. "You ain't heard from Lily by any chance, have you?"

"Nope." Not an ounce of feeling. Her ma didn't even lift her eyes from her task.

Honestly, Violet believed she'd get a letter before her folks ever would. She just wished they'd hear something. *Anything* to let them know Lily was all right.

Violet had taken all the coldness she could bear. She scooted her chair back and stood. "I hafta get home. We got our own apples to pick and peel."

"Fine. Give your in-laws my best."

Violet nodded and left. Her ma's *best* hadn't reared its head in a very long time.

Chapter 5

A stream of sunlight penetrated the thin curtain fabric and illuminated Lily's room. She'd hardly slept at all.

Arabelle had stayed in her room all day and night. She'd not come out for supper or to tell the children goodnight. They'd each taken a turn going into her room, but none of them stayed long. How their family could function this way was beyond Lily.

Though Mr. Jacobson had shown Lily how to tend his wife, he'd taken it upon himself to care for her the rest of the evening. Today, it would be Lily's responsibility. She didn't mind, but she had an abundance of tasks to accomplish, and she hoped she'd be able to manage them all.

The sound of a spoon clinking against a cup brought her upright in bed. She assumed Mr. Jacobson had also risen.

Lily quickly dressed. Her bedroom afforded her little space, but it was sufficient. Mr. Jacobson had told her that prior to her arrival they'd used it for storage. Her bed had been shoved against one wall. Aside from that, she had a single chair, a small nightstand, and a bureau, but no wardrobe. Since she owned only two dresses, she could easily make do. She kept the garments draped over the chair.

She shuffled through her knapsack and found her hairbrush, then drew it through her tangled mess. After a night of tossing about in bed, her hair had suffered. Once she'd smoothed it, she fashioned a loose braid. It would keep the long strands out of her face and not trouble her while she worked.

Her plain room needed color—or something to brighten it. For the time being, she opened the curtains completely to let the sunshine fully in.

She shut her eyes.

Lord, help me get through this day.

Regardless of her success, she had nowhere else to go.

She needed to write to Violet and tell her where she was living now. And even though she hadn't gotten over her ill feelings toward her folks, she'd pen a letter to them as well. Violet would no doubt tell them her news, yet Lily felt it best that it come directly from her. If she intended to heal and mend her life, she had to forgive her folks for sending her away.

She also wanted to write to the Waters and thank them for caring for her. Mrs. Gottlieb and Archibald, too.

"Mercy," she mumbled. "That's a lot a letters."

Fortunately, she had enough money remaining to afford postage. She still had to acquire something to write on, but assumed Mr. Jacobson's store would have proper paper.

With another quick prayer and a large breath, she left her room and made her way to the kitchen.

Mr. Jacobson was sitting at the table, sipping a cup of coffee. Levi cuddled against him.

"Good mornin'," Lily said.

"Good morning." Mr. Jacobson displayed his usual large smile. "You're up quite early. I hope I didn't wake you with all my knocking around in the kitchen."

"You didn't. I'm used to gettin' up at sunrise." She knelt beside him and Levi. "An' how are *you* this mornin'?" She set a hand on the boy's arm.

He shyly pulled away and buried his face in his pa's shirt.

She'd hoped he would open up to her a bit more. Not wanting to push him, she stood upright and stepped away.

"He's a daddy's boy," Mr. Jacobson said. "He was closer to his mother after he was born, but since the accident, he's latched onto me."

"*Literally.*" Lily let out a little laugh and smiled. "He must have an awful time when you leave for work."

The man nodded, then mouthed, *he usually cries*, while pretending to rub his eyes like a weeping child.

Lily understood perfectly.

"Do you drink coffee?" Mr. Jacobson asked.

"Sometimes. Truthfully, it sounds quite good right now."

"Please, help yourself. You'll find cups in the cupboard beside the stove." He gently patted Levi's back, all the while looking at her. "Once you get your coffee, why don't you join me here? We can chat."

She liked the idea. Not only did she enjoy talking to Mr. Jacobson, she had more questions than she could count.

Fortunately, in addition to the coffee cups, she found sugar. She couldn't bring herself to drink it black. With her beverage properly doctored, she took a seat across from Mr. Jacobson.

He peered over the rim of his cup. "Was your bed satisfactory?"

"Yes. Thank you."

"I want you to be comfortable here. It's important. I know we're asking a lot of you."

Lily sipped her hot drink. "I'll be fine. As I told you before, I'm grateful to be here."

"I plan to go by the telegraph office today and send word to Mr. and Mrs. Waters. I'll let them know you arrived safely."

"I appreciate it."

"Is there anyone else you'd like me to notify?"

The names of everyone Lily intended to write letters to spun through her mind. Yet, a telegram was impersonal and businesslike. "No. That should do. But I plan to *write* to quite a few folks. Could you bring home some paper an' envelopes for me? I have money."

"There's no need. I have everything you require here for letter-writing. And I'll happily post them for you."

"But—"

"No arguments. We never discussed pay. I don't expect you to work for free. I've never approved of slavery, and I won't start now."

"Slavery?" She sat back in her chair. "That's an odd thing to say. I'm here to help, an' I came here of my own free will. That's far from slavery."

"Maybe so. But I intend to pay you as well as provide room and board." He cleared his throat. "You'll have to forgive me. I still have many bitter feelings about the war."

Lily's questions tripled. "I reckon you saw an' heard a great deal at your store. What with folks comin' an' goin' all the time."

"Yes, I did. War is a terrible thing. The best day of all was when I heard Lee had surrendered. Of course, it was soon followed by the horrible news of Lincoln's death. Such a shameful tragedy on top of everything else the country had suffered."

She couldn't have heard him right. "I'm confused. Lincoln died *'fore* the war ended. I remember well when we was told. It was April of last year. It wasn't till May that we got word the war was over—a full month later."

Mr. Jacobson's brows creased. "No. That's not correct. I have the dates engrained in my mind. Lee surrendered April ninth, and Lincoln was assassinated by John Wilkes Booth on April fifteenth. Booth claimed he was avenging the South."

Lily's hands trembled as she set her cup on the table. "But—why didn't *we* know it? If the war ended in April—" Her stomach twisted into knots.

"Are you all right? You're pale."

She clutched her belly. "Soldiers came to the cove an' told us 'bout Lincoln, but they didn't say a word 'bout Lee's surrender. Wouldn't they a known?"

"Possibly. However, news never traveled well in the ranks. Or to remote areas like your cove. The rebels didn't *want* the war to end, so some refused to give up even when they learned of the surrender." He paused and glanced lovingly at his son, then met Lily's gaze. "I won't go into explicit detail, but some horrid things happened here in Asheville in late April of last year. Long after Lee's surrender. My store was plundered, and many people had their homes ransacked. Both sides did wretched, ugly things. I pray our country doesn't see such violence again. Ever."

The sadness in his eyes reflected her own feelings. Her thoughts spun out of control. Had Ableman purposely kept the truth from them?

If her family had known the war was over, Caleb could've stayed in the cove. Everything would've worked out as it should. She'd have the man she loved and the child she longed for.

Mr. Jacobson tapped his hand on the table in front of her. "You truly look ashen. I imagine you could use some food. Do you like oats?"

"Yessir." She doubted she could eat a bite, but the children would need a good breakfast. "Why don't you show me where they are, an' I'll fix them?" Keeping her hands busy might get her mind off the disturbing revelations, but part of her wanted to scream, or maybe just crumble to the floor and hover in a corner all day rehashing what could've been.

Mr. Jacobson's warm smile returned. He pointed to where the pots and pans were kept, then set Levi down and showed her the well-stocked pantry with all the dry storage. One thing was certain. No one in this house would ever go hungry.

Lily made herself at home in his kitchen and wasted no time getting the water ready for the oats. She had to let go of her anger. It wouldn't be right to reflect it on the children, or *anyone* here. *They'd* not done anything wrong to her.

Mr. Jacobson went back to his seat at the table. Levi immediately crawled onto his lap.

"I can see why it's hard for you to get things done 'round here." Lily glanced over her shoulder and pushed out a smile. "It's not easy workin' with a child attached to your body."

"True." Fortunately, he grinned.

Lily had to be careful and not so openly speak her mind. After all, she scarcely knew these folks.

She focused on stirring the oats. "I'm curious . . . how long have y'all lived in Asheville? I can tell by the way you talk that you're not from around here."

"We came from Montrose, Pennsylvania. It's in the northernmost part of the state."

Again, Lily looked back at him, smiled, and kept stirring.

"We arrived four years ago. Before we were blessed with Levi."

The boy's head popped up at the mention of his name. He grinned and patted his pa's face, but Lily wished the child would speak more.

"He truly is a blessin'. There's sumthin' special 'bout little boys." She whipped her head around in the opposite direction. Her face would surely show her pain and prompt questions she didn't want to answer.

"*Girls*, too. And mine should be getting out of bed."

"I can wake them when the oats are ready. They aren't too good if they sit on the stove for long."

"Thank you."

Lily set the spoon down, grabbed the coffeepot, and refilled his cup. "What possessed you to move here in the middle of the war?"

"Difficult circumstances." He nodded his thanks, then took a drink. "We'd gotten word that Arabelle's uncle Stanley had become ill. He owned the general store and needed help. He was childless and had named Arabelle as his heir. We moved here believing we'd step in and assist him, but arrived too late. He'd already passed. We were fortunate that the sheriff had locked up the place and kept an eye on it until our arrival. Otherwise, I imagine the store would've been emptied of its merchandise."

Lily held a hand to her heart. "I'm sorry 'bout his passin'. I shouldn't be pryin'."

"It's all right. You need to know about us, just as I hope to learn more about you."

That wouldn't be so easy. She'd rather keep him talking about himself. "How'd you manage keepin' yourself outta the war?"

His gaze shifted downward and his shoulders dropped.

"Never mind," she quickly said. "Forgive me for askin'."

"Money can do many things," he muttered.

Money.

When she'd lived in St. Louis, her life was so upside-down that she'd not given much thought to why so many of the young men hadn't served in the war. Maybe the wealthy fathers of men like Zachary and Archibald had ways of keeping them out of battle. Poor folks didn't have that luxury. No wonder her life there hadn't felt real. She'd been living in a protected bubble. Then again, she was certain there had to be men from that area who fought. The war touched every city. She probably didn't notice such things, because she hadn't been looking for them. Her mind had been preoccupied with what her aunt and uncle had planned for her future.

She scowled, recalling her life there.

"You must think I'm wretched," Mr. Jacobson whispered.

"Oh. *No.*" She rapidly shook her head. "Forgive me. I was thinkin' 'bout how things had been in St. Louis. I wasn't frownin' at *you.*"

His brows wove, then he took a quick drink. "I'm glad. You see—If I'd gone off to fight, I would've had to leave my family behind. They needed me. So, we did what we could to keep the soldiers happy by feeding them and providing other luxuries that weren't easy to come by. I'm not proud of the things I did, but I've suffered the most over what happened to my sister. I'm sure you recall that story."

Lily sadly nodded. His sister had been a prostitute in the war, who was killed by a drunk soldier. It didn't bother Lily that Mr. Jacobson was vague with details, but she was grateful he'd reached out to Water's Rest on behalf of his sister. Otherwise, Lily wouldn't have been given this opportunity.

"If I hadn't been so disgusted by Sarah's behavior," he went on, "I'd have sent her money to get her out of that mess. But I was arrogant and ashamed of her, so I turned my back." He sat a little taller. "Miss Larsen, learn from my mistake. I know you have family, and though I don't know your story, I pray that they will be loving and understanding. Because, no matter how bad anyone's behavior becomes, the heart seldom changes. No soul is ever truly lost. People stray. If you've not reached out to them, do so, before it's too late. I have no doubt they care more than you realize."

Her heart thumped hard. Though he'd spoken about *her*, she couldn't help but think about Lucas. "Are you sure you don't know my story? Cuz it feels like you're sayin' exactly what I need to hear."

Finally, he smiled again. "I'm glad. I doubt I'll ever overcome the guilt I feel for letting my sister down, but if I can help you, Sarah's loss will be easier to bear."

He tipped up his cup and rapidly drank the last of his coffee. "I should get to the store."

"Want me to wake the girls first, so you can tell them goodbye? An' what 'bout your wife?"

"I don't wish to wake Arabelle. She got almost no sleep last night. Oh—I forgot to mention the importance of her consumption of liquids. Encourage her to drink as much water as you can. It helps prevent infections." He looked at Lily with narrow eyes, questioning her understanding.

"Of course. That makes a lot a sense."

He cast a relieved smile. Lily assumed the thought of going into a detailed explanation made him uncomfortable. "As for the girls," he went on, "let's see how they do with you alone."

"But—" Lily gestured to the hot cereal. "What 'bout your breakfast?"

"Coffee is all I require." With a long, loud sigh, he stood and set Levi on the floor. "Now's the hard part," he whispered.

He strode across the room and grabbed his coat from the peg on the wall. The instant he threaded his arms into the sleeves, Levi let out a squall.

Lily hastened to the child's side. "Reckon *he'll* wake everyone." She stroked his head. "You'll be fine, sweetheart."

He paid her no mind and latched onto to his pa's legs, sobbing.

Mr. Jacobson bent to his level. "Miss Larsen will take good care of you. Papa will be home later." He kissed the boy's forehead, then stood erect.

Levi stretched his arms upward, all the while moving his legs as if it would help propel him into the man's embrace. Tears streamed down the child's red cheeks.

Mr. Jacobson opened the door and rushed out.

Levi's loud cry intensified.

"Shh . . ." Lily sat on her rump beside him. "Don't cry, Levi. I'm here for you."

He sniffled and sucked in air, all the while reaching out toward where his pa had been. The boy's lower lip vibrated out of control.

Lily wouldn't give up. She circled his legs with one arm and drew him nearer. "I'm gonna take of you. We'll have some oats with honey, an' later, I'll teach you a fun game."

Another sniffle. He blinked several times and pushed out more tears. However, his bawling ceased, and his arms dropped to his sides.

"Oats?" His tiny voice lifted her heart.

"That's right. An' we'll sweetin' 'em up with a big glob of honey. Won't that be good?"

With a single nod, he plopped into her lap.

Yes.

Footsteps came from behind her.

Opal approached, wearing a long nightgown. She rubbed her eyes and yawned. "How'd you get him to stop crying?"

"I reckon it was the promise of food." Smiling, Lily stroked Levi's tiny head, then reached out to Opal. "Are *you* hungry?"

"Uh-huh."

"Well, then. Let's wake up your sisters an' have some breakfast."

Opal smirked. "Good luck getting them outta bed. They sometimes act ugly in the morning."

Lily stood, and to her delight, Levi clung to her. "I have brothers who are impossible when they first wake up. They like to wrestle to work out their frustrations."

Opal giggled. "Winnie and Jenny don't wrestle. But, they *do* argue. Mother doesn't like it."

"Then, we'll work on that." Lily pondered her words. "You said *Jenny*. Is that what Genevieve prefers to be called?"

"Yep. I'm glad I'm Opal. Winnie and Jenny sounds silly. Don't you think so?"

"They rhyme." Lily grinned. "You all have lovely names." She returned with Levi to the kitchen, shifted him onto one hip, and pulled a highchair close to the table.

Opal took her own seat. "He usually eats while sitting on Father's lap."

Lily looked directly into Levi's wet eyes. "Are you a big boy?"

He bobbed his head.

"Can you show me?"

His little mouth screwed together and moved from side to side.

"You know how your pa sits in a chair by himself? Well, that's cuz he's a big boy, too. An' this here chair was made special for you, cuz it hoists you up high and you can sit at the table like your pa. Wanna try it?"

Another fast nod.

"Good." She planted him in the chair and positioned it at the table.

Instead of crying he beamed and sat tall. "Like Papa."

Joy pulsed through Lily. Her first accomplishment felt incredible. She spooned out some oats into bowls for Levi and Opal, then drizzled them with honey. Fortunately, Levi had mastered a spoon. Though he held it in his fist like a shovel, he managed to land the cereal in his mouth.

Opal's eyes opened wide. "I can't wait to tell Father that you got Levi in his highchair."

Lily simply smiled. She assumed they'd all have plenty to tell their pa when he got home from work. She only hoped it would all be good and not complaints about their demanding caregiver.

Chapter 6

Lily left Opal and Levi eating their breakfast, while she went to the older girls' room to wake them. On the way there, she paused and peeked in on Arabelle. She appeared to be fast asleep and unbothered by Levi's earlier outburst. She'd probably gotten used to it.

Lily chose to abide by Mr. Jacobson's request to let his wife sleep. At least for now. It would allow Lily to get all the children started on their day, and it would also afford her the time to get her mind right as to how she'd approach Arabelle. She didn't want to overwhelm the poor woman, but had every intention of proving to her that she was still capable of many things. Perhaps the experience Lily'd had with her pa had prepared her for this. From what Violet had told her, it had certainly helped *her* get Gideon on his feet again. Or, his *foot* as in his case.

Arabelle didn't have to walk to accomplish what she needed to do. Her wheelchair would suffice.

Lily rapped lightly on the girls' door before pushing it open. Memories of all the years she'd shared a room with Violet came to mind. However, unlike them, these two sisters didn't share the same bed. They each had their own.

Their bedroom was nothing like the storage space that had been converted for Lily. This one had been lavishly decorated.

Frills and lace abounded. The walls were papered with a floral print similar to the one that had been in Lily's room in St. Louis. But this pattern was lighter in color. It had soft pink roses intermingled with white daisies.

The girls' beds had sheer canopies and more than enough pillows. Their small bodies had been swallowed up in blankets. They both lay utterly still and looked quite warm and cozy.

Lily was about to change that.

No matter how pretty the area had been made to be, all the fineries were overshadowed with clutter. Lily stepped over a mound of clothes that had been left in the middle of the floor. Her foot landed on something small and hard. She bent down and picked up a miniature porcelain sofa.

She carefully examined the thing, fortunately finding it undamaged. The lovely item should be on a display shelf, but she assumed it was one of their toys. She spotted a two-story dollhouse covered partially by a towel. Amidst other pieces of discarded this and that, she noticed several dolls' heads poking out. Their wide eyes looked like they desperately cried for rescue.

She would've laughed if the situation wasn't so dismal.

She loudly cleared her throat, but it did no good. The girls didn't budge.

"Winnie." Lily kept her voice kind, but stern. "Jenny. Breakfast is ready. Y'all need to get up an' eat."

Winnie's blanket inched away from her face. "I'm too tired. I wanna sleep longer."

"Me, too," Jenny mumbled.

Lily carefully crossed the room, pulled each canopy to the side, then perched on the edge of Jenny's bed. "You can both sleep more t'night. We got lots to do today, an' the best way to start is by eatin' sumthin' that'll stick to your bones." She patted the blanket close to where Jenny lay. "C'mon, now. Wake up."

"But we *always* sleep late. We never get up till the church woman comes."

"The church women won't be comin' no more." Lily sat tall. "*I'm* carin' for you now, an' things are gonna be different."

Winnie sat up and folded her arms across her chest. "*How* different?"

Jenny also wiggled into an upright position. "Yes. How different, Miss Larsen?" She yawned and stretched.

Lily smiled at each girl in turn. "Remember when I told you I'd need your help to find my way 'round here?"

They both nodded.

"Part of that includes gettin' things in order. In case you haven't noticed, the house is a mess. Your room alone looks like it was hit by a tornado. I wasn't hired to be a maid, I was brought here to care for y'all. I don't mind cleanin' the house, but it's *your* home an' you need to do your part. Understand?"

Jenny gulped. "You mean, you're gonna make us *work*?" She grimaced when she said the word.

Lily smiled. "I've never thought of household chores as work. They're more of a responsibility. 'Sides, won't it be nice havin' things clean an' orderly?"

Jenny primly folded her hands atop the blankets. "Mother says it's more important to use our imaginations and do creative things."

"And play outside in the sunshine," Winnie added. "There's a tree behind our house where I built a fort. We like to go there and pretend we're on adventures."

"I'd like you to show it to me," Lily said. "*After* we finish all our tasks on the inside. Once chores are done, there'll be plenty a time for play. I promised Levi I'd teach him a game my family enjoys."

Winnie threw back her covers and swung her legs over the side of her bed. "You know some games?"

"Yep. An' I also know ways to make chores fun, too."

Jenny sighed and got out from beneath her blankets. "I don't see how."

Lily ran her hand over Jenny's long hair. "Give me a chance to show you." Again, she studied both girls' expressions. They seemed to be intrigued and not so negative anymore. "You love your folks, don't you?"

"Uh-huh," Jenny said.

"Of course, we do," Winnie added.

"Then, let's surprise 'em an' fix up the house so beautiful that when your pa gets home from work, he'll think he's come to the wrong place."

The girls giggled.

"What about our mother?" Winnie asked. "She won't know the difference, because she doesn't come out of her room."

Lily stood. "I plan to change that. Your ma could use a bit of sunshine herself."

Jenny got to her feet and took hold of Lily's arm. "She won't leave her bed. She says she can't."

"Hasn't she ever gotten out in the wheelchair?"

Both girls frowned and shook their heads.

"If it was me," Lily said. "I'd hate bein' cooped up inside all the time." Her mind spun. "How long ago was her accident?"

"March," Winnie said. "Right before Easter. It was the first time Mother didn't go to church on Easter Sunday. Everyone has been understanding, but whenever we go without her, they ask Father when she's coming back. He always says, *hopefully soon*."

"But he knows it's not true," Jenny quickly said. "She'll *never* go. Father has started to make excuses why *we* can't go to church. It makes him sad to be there without Mother."

"I understand." Lily gave Jenny's hand a squeeze. "Maybe we can change that, too."

They eyed her like they thought she was crazy. And maybe she was. But Lily was determined to make a difference. "All right. Let's go eat some oatmeal, then we'll get y'all dressed. Do you have sumthin' less fancy to wear than what you had on yesterday?"

"Something to *work* in?" Winnie asked.

Lily pinched her lips together. "Sumthin' you won't mind gettin' dirty. An' preferably without lace."

Jenny whimpered. "I *like* lace."

"C'mon," Lily put an arm around her shoulder, then reached for Winnie's hand. "Breakfast first. I promise you'll feel better once you've eaten."

She guided them to the table where they joined Opal and Levi.

Levi lifted his bowl. "More?"

Lily happily obliged him, and after she got all the children eating their breakfast, she spooned some oats into a bowl for Arabelle.

"Y'all keep eatin', I'm gonna take this to your ma."

"Isn't it too early to wake her up?" Winnie asked.

Lily pulled her shoulders back. "Maybe earlier than usual, but if she doesn't sleep all day, I reckon she'll sleep better at night."

Jenny nudged her older sister. "She really *is* doing things different."

Lily jutted her chin and headed for Arabelle's room.

Though the woman wasn't snoring, she breathed slow, loud, and steady, and her eyes were shut tight. Lily had no doubt that she was in a deep sleep.

A bed tray had been placed atop the bureau, so Lily set the oats on it, then parted the curtains to let in some light.

"Arabelle?" Lily inched close to the bed. "I brought breakfast."

The woman's shoulders jerked and her eyes fluttered open. "Lily? Why'd you wake me?"

"You need to eat, ma'am, an' I didn't want the oats to overcook."

"I'm not hungry." She closed her lids and burrowed her head deeper into the pillow.

"You surely must be." Lily wouldn't give up. "You ate scarcely anythin' last night. Can't you at least *try* to eat?"

"Leave me be. Please? And shut the drapes. The light hurts my eyes."

Though she hesitated for a moment, Lily did as she asked.

"Thank you." Arabelle looked directly at her. "Because you're just now learning our ways, I won't fault you this morning. I'll call for you when I wake. And when I do, your first concern every morning is to change me. Food comes later."

"Yes'm."

With a heavy heart, Lily grabbed the bowl of cereal and left Arabelle's room, closing the door behind her. She took a seat at the table with the children and ate the oats herself. She'd need her strength. It was going to be a very long day.

Winnie leaned across the table. "I tried to warn you that it was too early. None of us have ever been up this soon." She sat straight and kept eating.

Lily considered her words. "Levi was up with your pa, an' I reckon he does that every mornin'. So, who's been tendin' him after your pa goes to work?"

"Me," Opal said. "Levi an' I share a room. Most mornings he cries for a long time after Father leaves, then comes and crawls in bed with me. He usually cries himself to sleep."

"That's no way to tend a baby," Lily mumbled, but immediately regretted saying it. Her words would very well be repeated by one of the children to their folks.

"He's not a baby," Jenny said. "He's been out of diapers for over a year. Good thing, too. Mrs. Wood sometimes complains about the soiled cloths from our *mother's* accidents."

"Hush, Jenny." Winnie shoved against her shoulder with one hand. "We're not supposed to talk about that."

Jenny stared at the table, frowning.

"Who's Mrs. Wood?" Lily asked.

Winnie sat tall. "She's a widow woman who does our laundry."

"You don't wash your own clothes?"

Winnie's eyes drew open wide. "Of course not. We'd surely ruin them. Mrs. Wood takes extra care of all our fine things. She doesn't mind the lacy dresses so much, and Father pays her for each individual item she launders. Jenny shouldn't have mentioned the soiled cloths. We were told to keep that to ourselves." She crinkled her nose at her sister, and Jenny replied by sticking out her tongue.

"That's enough a that, girls," Lily scolded. "Truthfully, I think we *should* talk 'bout it. Do y'all understand why your ma has *accidents*?" She looked from face to face. The girls nodded, but Levi paid her no mind. Of course, she didn't expect him to comprehend the subject matter.

"Father says it's private," Winnie said.

"Yes, it is. But you're her children, an' her family. We can talk 'bout anythin' we want inside these walls. I may not be related, but I was brought here to help, so I'm kinda like family now, too. Your ma's condition is very serious. You know she won't ever walk again, right?"

The girls slowly bobbed their heads.

"An' yes, she has accidents like a baby. But that means we gotta give her extra special care." She turned to Winnie. "Since you're the oldest, did you ever change Levi when he was still in diapers?"

"Yes. I didn't like it, but Mother told me that every girl should know how to tend babies, so when I have my own, I'll know what to do.

"That's right. Did you ever see Levi get a rash, if he wasn't changed right away?"

"A couple times. But Mother tried very hard to keep him clean." She dropped her hands into her lap and lowered her head. "She was a good mother. And she used to laugh a lot." Slowly, she lifted her tear-filled eyes. "It's not fair what happened to her."

Lily stood and went to the girl's side, then squatted down and put an arm around her. "You're right, it's not fair. But your ma was blessed with all a you. If we work together, I know we can get her laughin' again."

Droplets trickled down Winnie's cheeks. "You promise?"

Lily kissed her forehead. "I'll do all I can to make it happen. But I can't without every one a you."

"*I* wanna help," Jenny said.

"Me, too," Opal chimed in.

"Good." Lily faced Winnie. "Can I count on you?"

She sniffled and nodded. "I'm just scared. I know it won't ever be the way it was, but I don't like the way it is now. Show us what to do. I overheard Father call you an angel. If you can make our mother happy again, then I'll believe it."

Lily wiped tears from Winnie's face. "I'm a regular person like you. But I know I can help." She smiled and rose. "Finish your cereal, then we have work to do."

Jenny giggled. "You mean, *responsibilities*?"

Lily couldn't help but laugh with her. "That's right. Least I know you got good ears."

Levi put both hands to the sides of his head. "Ears."

"That's right, sweetheart." Lily grabbed a rag to clean off his oatmeal-covered face. "Those are your ears."

The children filled her with more hope than ever.

With their help, she was determined to bring the entire family back to life again.

Chapter 7

Violet wanted to return home as fast as she could and distance herself from her ma, so she pushed Stardust hard.

For months, Violet had been trying to forgive the woman for sending Lily away, but her ma's treatment of Noah made it impossible. The child needed his real ma and all the love that Lily could give him.

When she thought about how unconcerned her ma seemed regarding Lily's whereabouts, it infuriated her even more. Her ma obviously didn't care about *anyone* any longer.

Violet gripped the saddle horn so tight it made her hands hurt. Even so, she dug her heels into the horse's sides. "C'mon Stardust, show me how fast you can run!" She'd become an accomplished rider, but rarely let the mare run free. When Stardust broke into a wild gallop, Violet hung on for dear life.

The heavy pounding of Stardust's hooves matched the angry rhythm of Violet's heart. With every hard-thumping footfall against the dirt road, she internally cursed. Something she'd never openly do.

She steered the eager horse to the pasture, eased her to a stop, then leaned forward and hugged her sweaty neck. "Good girl. Sorry I took out some a my frustrations on *you*." She gave her a pat and dismounted.

With a huff, she glanced at the mare's saddle, but didn't care to bother with it at the moment. The horse trotted off and joined two others in the field. Stardust tossed her mane, then lowered her head to the grass. They all looked serene, casually grazing.

Violet, however, was ready to spit nails.

She turned on her heels and marched in the opposite direction. She hoped to find Gideon in the barn. If she didn't talk about what had happened with her ma, she might explode.

To her dismay, she found him by the woodshed, chopping wood. Her stomach roiled for a different reason. Though he swore he could capably swing the axe and keep his balance—even teetering on a crutch—she feared he'd hurt himself.

"Gideon!"

He whipped around and faced her. "Don't start on me, Violet. I told you I can manage this."

"It's not that." She hurried to his side. "Well, it still bothers me, but that's not what's irritatin' me right this minute."

He laughed and leaned the axe against the woodpile. "What is, then?"

She erupted into unexpected tears. Anger had pushed her to her limit. "I didn't see Noah. Ma has Mrs. Henderson tendin' him. I told Ma she shoulda brung him here, but she said I was gettin' too close to Noah an' confusin' him." She latched onto her husband and buried her face against his neck. "It ain't right!"

"Don't cry, sweetheart." He threaded his fingers into her hair and gently pulled them through.

The sensation he created slightly calmed her, but her heart continued to pound. "I love that baby. Ma don't care one bit about him." She lifted her head to look Gideon in the eyes. "I reckon she resents him. He's a reminder of the shame Lily brought on the family. But Noah's just a little baby. It ain't his fault."

Gideon guided her to a pair of upturned logs and they both sat. He grabbed hold of her hands. "Mrs. Henderson is a kind woman. She'll take good care a Noah."

"But she ain't his kin. I *am*. If Ma don't wanna look after him, *I* should. Noah needs his family."

Gideon tenderly stroked her skin. "I know how much you love him, but your ma's right. He ain't yours. Since your folks told everyone in the cove that he's theirs, it's up to them to decide what's best for the boy."

"But I promised Lily—"

"I know. You swore to keep an eye on him. Your ma ain't makin' it easy. I'm sure once winter comes, they'll keep Noah with them at the cabin, then maybe if the snow ain't too deep, you can visit him some."

"What if they decide to give him up to the Hendersons?"

"They won't." He patted the top of her hand. "It would hurt their reputation—sumthin' they've been tryin' awful hard to keep upstandin'. Maybe this was the first time they took him there. I doubt your folks would send him away a lot."

"I hope you're right. But the way Ma talked, I know she don't want him with her. If Lily knew how she treated him, it would break her heart."

"Then don't tell her. I know you like to write an' share all we got goin' on, but some things are best left unsaid. I'm sure Lily has enough to worry 'bout right now."

Violet shut her eyes and rested her head on her husband's shoulder. "You're right. 'Sides, I don't even know where she's gone. What if she's hurt? Or sick? Not knowin' is tearin' me up inside. I keep hopin' to hear from her."

"You will. Have you forgotten how strong an' capable she is? Lily knows how to take care a herself better than most folks. She's probably gettin' settled in somewhere. I'm sure she'll have lots to tell."

"Thank you for sayin' that." She squeezed him tight. "I needed to hear it. If only she'd come back to the cove." She huffed out a large burst of air, released him, and dried her tears with the sleeve of her dress. Lately, her emotions had been up and down like a bird in flight.

"Ever thought a talkin' to your pa 'bout how you're feelin'? You know—'bout Noah *an'* Lily. Seems he's a mite more reasonable than your ma."

"He used to not be reasonable at all. But he's been better since he stopped tippin' the jug. If it weren't for Pa, my folks never woulda come to our weddin' reception." The terrible memory worsened her already dismal mood. Her ma had behaved horribly that day.

"Why don't you go talk to him? I can almost guarantee *he's* worried 'bout Lily. An' maybe you can get a sense of his feelin's for the boy. He might even tell you how often Mrs. Henderson watches him."

Violet stared into nothingness pondering the idea. She had to do *something* about it or she'd keep losing sleep from worry. She blinked a few times, then focused solely on her husband's caring face. "I'll wait a few days to calm down first. I'm afraid if I go back there now an' Noah's still gone, I might say sumthin' I'll regret."

"I reckon there's a lot a things need sayin'. But, you're right. It's not smart to lash out in anger." Gideon nodded toward the cabin. "Why don't you go see Ma, while I finish up here? Maybe she can cheer you up. She enjoys havin' you to talk to, an' you won't have to watch me cut wood. When I'm done, I'll come fetch you, an' we'll go pick some apples."

"All right. I certainly like talkin' to your ma, more so than my own. Is it odd to prefer your in-law's company?" Simply thinking about Gideon's kind ma improved Violet's mood.

"Maybe. But I'm glad you like my folks."

"Actually . . ." Violet gazed upward. "I don't."

"What?" Gideon's mouth dropped wide open.

Violet giggled. "I *love* them, silly man." She kissed him squarely on the lips. "I'll leave you to your choppin'. Promise you'll be careful with that axe, all right?"

"I will. Winter's comin'. We gotta get as much wood as we can."

She grinned. "An' plenty a snugglin'." As she strode away, she glanced over her shoulder with a more enticing smile. It would give him something to think about until they were together again. And when she was alone with him, no bad thoughts ever crept in. Nights cuddled against him had become her favorite time of every day.

Her heart skipped with a happier beat. She never stopped being amazed at the difference true love had made in her life.

* * *

Gideon stood completely still and watched his wife walk away. Of course, his heart thumped hard. The look she gave him boiled his blood.

He was glad he'd lifted her spirits, but hated that he'd added to her troubles, worrying over his capability to chop wood. After all, she'd been the one who'd told him he could do most anything and got him working again.

It wasn't easy to balance himself while trying to split the logs, but he'd figured out a way to squeeze the crutch into his armpit to keep him upright. He swung the axe capably with his right arm, while steadying himself with the left. It had taken a while to master the task, but once he'd accomplished it, overcoming the hardship gave him a sense of pride.

Violet had been a lot more emotional recently, but she had every right to be upset about Noah. He'd never understand Mrs. Larsen.

He recalled how different the woman had been when he and Violet were younger. Her ma had smiled more and seemed pleasant. She hadn't been overly friendly to him, but then again, why would she have paid any mind to a boy?

Seems she still don't wanna give boys no attention.

He decided to stop thinking about Violet's ma and concentrate on his wife. Someone much more pleasant.

If he didn't have so many chores, he'd take Violet in the wagon and go pay the Hendersons a visit. If she could see Noah and be reassured he was fine, it would make her feel a lot better. But there weren't enough hours in a day to work *and* call on neighbors.

He stacked the wood, then put the axe in its place with the other tools in the barn and headed for the cabin. They had apples to pick.

* * *

Gideon squinted into the sunlight. "You sure you can manage?"

Violet grabbed hold of the tree limb and hoisted herself up. "Long as I don't hafta go too high. The boys always got the apples at the top a the trees. I usually just waited below an' caught 'em."

"I hate you hafta climb at all." He scratched the back of his head. "Reckon I could *try.*"

She perched on the limb and smoothed her skirt. "I'm fine. It'd be hard for you to get up here."

"Well . . . be careful." He hated his limitations. Sometimes, he wished he would've given the fake leg a better try. Maybe if he'd spent more time working it, it would've stopped hurting.

Violet held onto the limb with one hand and plucked apples with the other. "Lily would die if she saw me up here. I wouldn't a done anythin' like this years ago."

Gideon stood below her and caught the fruit as she dropped it down. He then tossed it into a bucket beside his foot. "What made you decide to do it now?"

She grabbed onto the tree with both hands and stared down at him. "Necessity."

Her simple word stabbed deep. "Cuz *I* can't, right?" He frowned and turned away.

"Don't go startin' that now." She let out a little growl. "Gideon, look at me!"

He did as she asked, but felt no better.

Her eyes narrowed. "I wasn't sayin' it as a bad thing. You've made me a better person. I used to let Lily do everythin', an' I just sat back not wantin' to get my hands dirty. But now, I *like* doin' things like this." She waved in the air, gesturing to the tree. Her body teetered.

"Careful, Violet!"

She giggled and steadied herself. "I told you, I'm *fine*."

"It ain't funny. I don't know what I'd do if sumthin' bad happened to you." He swallowed the lump in his throat. "You're everythin' to me."

She inched across the limb, then repositioned herself on another branch. "You, too." Her humor vanished and she cast one of her most beautiful smiles. "I swear I'll do all I can to keep from fallin'. I won't go any higher. There's plenty of other trees to pick from. We can head on up the road, soon as I get these here." She nabbed a large apple, then tossed it to him.

He caught it with one hand. "I'll be glad when you're on the ground again."

She cleared all the fruit within reach, then eased down the trunk of the tree. "Better?" With pursed lips, she sauntered close.

"Much." He pulled her against his chest and kissed her perfect mouth.

A happy-sounding sigh escaped her. "I like it better on the ground, too." She gave him a quick peck. "I'll put this bucket in the wagon, then we can head up the road."

"I'll help." He grabbed one handle, and she took the other. Being nearly full, the heavy pale would've been difficult for her to manage.

They hoisted it into the wagon, then took their seats. Violet wiggled across, till her body butted against his. "I'm glad you hitched up Stardust. She likes bein' out an' about. Did I tell you how fast she ran earlier?"

He held the reins, but didn't budge the wagon from its place. He turned in the seat to face her. "I ain't never seen you ride her fast. Why did ya?"

She worked her lower lip with her teeth. "Cuz I was mad at my ma. Reckon I took it out on Stardust. But it felt incredible racin' in the wind. There's nothin' like it."

"But if she'd lost her footin'—what then?"

Violet tapped his leg. "You worry too much. I'm a good rider, an' Stardust is gentle. You'd know that yourself if you'd ever get on her back. She rides fast an' smooth, an'—"

"An' you can stop right there." He faced forward. "Don't *ever* expect me to ride her—or *any* horse. How many times do I gotta tell you?" He snapped the reins.

Violet's arms flailed, and she grabbed onto the seat. "Goodness, you got a temper." She huffed and sat rigid. "I know you've told me many times, but *I'm* tellin' *you*—your thighs are plenty strong enough to keep you seated on a horse. Trust me on that." With a quick single nod, she looked away.

He gulped, understanding her implication. "Sorry I get so ill." Yes, he had an awful temper, but he'd been trying to control it. She was the last person he'd ever want to upset. "Forgive me?" He lightly rubbed her leg.

She stared at his hand for a moment, then her body relaxed. "Course I do." She held his hand in her own and caressed his fingers with her thumb. "I know you well an' I understand some things scare you. I'd think swingin' a sharp axe would be harder than ridin' a horse. But I won't pester you again 'bout it. The horse ridin', that is. I'll try an' be more sensitive."

"I don't wanna break my neck. That's all. I do that, an' I *will* be worthless."

She rested her head on his shoulder. "You won't ever be worthless to me."

He couldn't help but smile. Violet had a way of ruffling his feathers, but she definitely brought out the best in him.

He parked the wagon below another large apple tree, but didn't move to get out. Instead, he pressed his hand to her belly. "You always ask me to be careful with the axe, an' I am. Will you promise *me* sumthin'?"

She looked into his eyes. "Course. What is it?"

He moved his hand in slow circles over her stomach. "Once you're with child, don't be climbin' no trees, an' please don't let Stardust run when you ride her. I want you an' our baby safe. All right?"

Her eyes misted over. "I promise."

They kissed, then kissed some more. It wasn't until Stardust whinnied that Gideon pulled away from Violet and remembered where they were.

He laughed. "Apples . . ." he muttered.

"Yep." Violet stood, then hopped from the wagon.

Gideon got out a lot slower, but she had him feeling light as air.

Apples now.

Babies later.

Chapter 8

Once Rebecca's mother-in-law had left for home, Rebecca decided to do what she did best. Since it was apple season, she had plenty for pies.

She proficiently crimped the edges. Humming a made-up tune, she put her signature cut on the upper crust. The shape of three perfect leaves at the center and tiny little slits all the way around. To make it extra tasty, she brushed melted butter over the top, then sprinkled it with sugar.

She smiled, just thinking about the expression on Caleb's face when he'd bite into the delicious dessert.

Their small oven was sufficient for a single pie, but she missed the large capacity of the ovens at the hotel. Truthfully, she missed many things about Iverson's—like having a maid to clean up after them and a cook to prepare every meal.

Her life would be a great deal more enjoyable if she only had to worry about pleasing her husband and raising their children.

Child.

The thought doused her good mood. She felt like a failure, unable to conceive again. It made no sense whatsoever. With Abraham, it had been easy.

The back door burst open. Caleb strode in wearing his usual straw hat and not-so-common large grin. "You need to come an' see what I built!"

She pressed her fingers to her lips. "Shh. Avery's nappin'."

He covered his mouth with one hand. "Sorry," he whispered.

An unpleasant odor surrounded her. She stepped closer to her husband and sniffed. "What've you been into? Manure?"

"Well . . . I ain't been *in* it, but I've been shovelin' it."

She waved a hand in front of her nose. "I can tell. Go back outside, an' I'll come see what it is you want to show me. Then, you best be takin' a bath."

"All right." His grin returned. "I think you're gonna like what I done." His eyes widened and he peered beyond her. "Apple pie?"

"Yep. I need to put it in the oven." She nudged him toward the door. "Go on now. I'll be right there."

He rubbed his hands together and wiggled his brows. "I love your pie."

"I know." She pointed outside.

Chuckling, he left.

She opened the oven door and stuck the pie in. Though she'd take the time to see what Caleb was so excited about, she had to be sure she got back to the house before the pie burned. She'd let it happen once before. A horrible memory.

Before going outside, she peeked in at Avery. Her sweet baby girl soundly slept.

Rebecca tiptoed down the hallway and went to find Caleb.

It wasn't hard. He was waiting right outside the back door. He took her hand and guided her to the tall oak beside the house. Because he acted so happy, she didn't care to dampen his mood by fussing about his smell. She held her breath as they walked.

Caleb beamed and pointed. "I made sure it's good an' secure. It held me, so I know it'll hold you. Avery, too."

"A swing?" The wood seat had been suspended from ropes tied in large knots to a limb of the tree.

"Yep. Remember how we used to swing at your folks' place? I always liked the way your hair flew behind you."

"You did?"

"Uh-huh." He smoothed his hand down her long locks. "You looked so beautiful. Happy, too." He leaned down and kissed her forehead, then gestured toward the seat. "Try it out."

His kind action and eagerness moved her. She completely disregarded his odor and went to the swing.

Before sitting, she tugged on the ropes.

Caleb cocked his head to one side. "Don't you trust me?"

"I trust *you*, but those knots could come untied."

"They won't. I know how to secure 'em just right."

She eased onto the swing, then grabbed hold of the ropes and pushed off with her feet. Glorious memories filled her mind. Her pa loved to push her on the swing. She'd always cry out, *higher, pa, higher!*

Newer memories came forward. Abraham and Caleb taking turns with her on the swing. Each seeing how high they could go. Her pa eventually put up two swings, though there should've been three. The three of them were inseparable.

She closed her eyes and leaned back. As she moved forward, her hair fluttered behind her, then as the swing went backward, it fell to her shoulders.

"Just like I recollect," Caleb said. "You like it?"

"I *love* it. What made you think to do it?"

"I wanted to make sumthin' Avery could enjoy, but when I started fixin' it, I figgered you'd have as much fun as her. By the look on your face, maybe more."

Rebecca pumped her legs to go faster. "Avery's too little to get on by herself. We'll have to sit with her for the time bein'."

"Looks like you won't mind." He chuckled. "Least I'll know where to find you if you ain't in the house."

She loved the sensation of floating on air.

The pie!

She eased the swing to a stop and jumped off. "Your dessert will burn, if I don't go back inside."

Caleb wrapped his arms around her. "Are you happy?"

"Yes. This is the nicest thing you've done for us. Thank you."

His eyes penetrated deep into hers. "I love you, Becca."

This was exactly how she'd wanted their life. To simply be in love and happy. "I love you, too."

He gave her a kiss she'd never forget. Her feet nearly lifted from the ground. When they separated, her heart thumped hard. "Oh, my, Caleb."

Again, he jiggled his brows.

She swatted his arm. "I need to get to that apple pie before it's black an' crispy."

"When can I have some?"

His playful expression told her he wasn't talking about the pie. "After supper." Her lips twitched into a grin. "You're shameful, Caleb Henry. I know what you're thinkin'."

"That means you're thinkin' it, too."

She giggled, lifted her skirt to keep from stumbling, and ran to the house.

* * *

Caleb sat on the swing and pushed off with his feet. He couldn't stop smiling. Seeing Rebecca so happy made his hard work worthwhile.

At times, he doubted she understood how difficult it was to keep the farm going. Sure, he smelled like manure, but only because they had horses and cows that had to be cleaned up after.

Since his wife rarely stepped foot outside, she couldn't possibly know what he did all day.

Someone like Lily, on the other hand, would know exactly how he spent his time.

He wished he could let go of her memory, but at least he'd learned how to love Rebecca. And, as time went on, he thought of Lily less and less.

Avery held most of his attention. Each little thing she did enthralled him. She seemed to learn something new every day. How could anyone *not* find that captivating?

The ropes creaked as he moved back and forth. He glanced upward to make sure the knots held firm. And of course, they did. Years ago, his pa had taught him how to tie an efficient knot.

At times like this, he missed the man more than ever. If only he'd been able to tell him goodbye.

He'd learned everything he knew from his pa. How to farm. How to manage money. And even how to treat women kindly. It would've been interesting to know what kind of advice his pa would've given him regarding Lily. Likely a lot different than what Caleb had gotten from his ma.

Caleb hoped that when he had a son, he could pass on the same kind of knowledge his pa had bestowed on him.

Noah.

No matter how hard he tried, he couldn't wash away the possibility of already having a son. He shut his eyes and let the wind cool his face. He'd do better if he'd focus on the positive things in his life. Specifically, his wife and daughter. As his ma always told him, they were what truly mattered.

Fall wasn't the smartest season of the year to put up a swing. But he'd followed his instincts regardless. Rebecca's reaction affirmed he'd done well.

The sun was nowhere close to setting and he had lots more work to do before taking the requested bath.

Part of him wanted to stay right where he was and forget work for a while, but his good senses took over.

While still high in the air, he let go of the ropes and jumped from the swing. He landed solidly on his feet, grinning. It had taken him many tries as a boy to master that skill. Not to mention, lots of bruises and scraped knees.

He headed to the barn. He'd not finished with the manure, so he grabbed the shovel and got busy. He had quite a while before Rebecca would call him in for supper.

Fortunately, all the corn had been harvested, and the wheat sown. Even so, his work was never done. With winter coming, he had to be sure there was plenty of feed for the livestock, wood for the house, and food for their own purpose. He also needed to give the house a good go-over to make certain all the cracks in the walls were filled and the roof could withstand heavy snow.

The same thing I done for the Larsens.

He stopped what he'd been doing, rested a hand atop the shovel, and stared toward the mountains. They called to him.

The answer to every question that plagued his mind lay in the cove.

His heart beat faster with every passing second.

If he ever wanted peace, he had to know.

Come spring, nothing would stop him from taking that three-day ride. He'd have to figure out an excuse to give Rebecca, but he had plenty of time to ponder it. His ma would surely give him grief if she knew where he planned to go.

Maybe it would be best to lie and say he was going someplace else. Somewhere like Asheville. It wasn't unheard of. He could tell them he needed supplies for the farm that he couldn't get in Waynesville.

He started shoveling again. Though he hated to lie, if he wanted to save himself from his ma's ranting, he wouldn't have a choice.

It seemed strange to have to use a lie to uncover the truth, but he'd do whatever it took.

The sun dipped low on the horizon by the time he finished all his chores and headed to the house.

When he walked in, he discovered that Rebecca had been just as busy as him. A fine-smelling supper simmered on the stove. The nicely browned apple pie rested on the countertop. And in the corner of the room, Rebecca had a tub of water already waiting for him. Steam rose from the metal vessel.

Rebecca sauntered up to him, but stopped before getting real close. "Perfect timin'." She held her nose with the tips of her fingers on one hand, and pointed to the tub with the other.

Avery toddled over to him. She, too, stopped and wrinkled her nose. "Pa 'tinks."

"Yes, he does." Rebecca scooped her up. "Let's you an' me go outside an' swing, while your pa takes a bath." She looked directly at Caleb. "Do you mind?"

"Course not. It's what I made it for."

"I got stew simmerin'. It'll be fine on the stove till you're ready to eat." She cuddled Avery close. "I can't wait to show her the swing."

"You go on then. I'll clean up an' make you both happier."

Rebecca inched closer to him. "I *am* happy as can be." She gave him a fast peck, then hastened out the door.

Caleb stripped bare and eased into the tub. The warm water embraced his body and soothed his aching muscles.

If this was all the life he knew, he'd be content.

Yet knowing all he did, kept him far from it.

Chapter 9

It took Lily a while to dig through all the children's clothes to find them proper attire for cleaning the house. Almost everything the girls owned had lace. She finally found some plain cotton dresses that had been tucked away at the bottom of a bureau drawer.

Jenny wrinkled her nose at the fabric, but Lily insisted she put on the beige dress.

Winnie acted more agreeable and readily donned her blue garment. "This is more comfortable than those other dresses." She turned sideways and looked at herself in a full-length mirror. "One day, I hope girls will be allowed to wear pants like boys. It would be much easier to climb trees."

Jenny rolled her eyes. "There she goes again. I told you we should call her *Fred*."

Winnie stomped her foot. "Don't say that!"

"Girls!" Lily clapped her hands a single time. "Behave yourselves." She turned to Jenny. "Your sister was statin' an opinion. That doesn't mean she *wants* to be boy. There's no need to tease her."

"But it's improper for a girl to talk about wearing pants." Jenny's brows dipped low. "Isn't it?"

"As I said earlier, we're all family, an' we should be able to comfortably talk 'bout anythin'." She took Jenny's hand. "I'm not angry with either of you, but you've got to start tryin' harder to get along an' not argue. If we wanna help your ma, we gotta keep the house peaceful. All right?"

Jenny lowered her eyes and nodded. "Sorry."

"It's fine. Now, let's get Opal an' Levi dressed an' get busy."

The younger children were even easier to please. Of course, at Levi's age, clothes weren't the least bit important. Lily recalled that her little brothers always preferred to run around in next-to-nothing when the weather permitted. Every memory such as that tugged at the hole in her heart. At least her newfound family helped fill part of the emptiness.

Lily found a large basket in the pantry. She set it in the middle of the living room floor. "I want all of you to go through the house an' find every stray item of clothin' an' any dirty towels or beddin'. Bring it all in here an' put it in this basket."

Opal sniggered. "It won't fit. There's too much."

"Then stuff what you can inside an' put the rest on the floor next to it. While y'all do that, I'm gonna tend your ma." Lily faced Winnie. "I'm countin' on *you* to keep an eye on Levi."

"Yes'm."

"Good girl. Be sure y'all count each item you bring. We'll see who gathers the most."

Winnie grinned. "That sounds like a game."

"Yep. So, get goin' an' we'll see who wins."

Lily didn't have to give them any more encouragement. All three girls headed off to hunt for dirty laundry. Winnie tugged on Levi's hand, and he laughed as they ran off together.

Now came the hard part.

Earlier, Lily hadn't made a good impression on Arabelle, but she hoped to improve the woman's opinion of her.

Before going to her room, Lily heated some water and filled the large pan she'd used before. She gathered a few clean rags and a dose of bravery and made her way to Arabelle's bedside. This time, she found that her eyes were wide open.

"Good mornin'," Lily said as sweetly as she could.

Arabelle turned her head. "I didn't call for you."

"But you're awake. I'm sure you need changin'. The sooner I do it, the better you'll be."

"Go on then. Do what you must."

Arabelle shut her eyes and kept her head turned away from Lily.

The children's giggles seeped into the bedroom, but their ma showed no reaction. It seemed she had no interest whatsoever in what they might be doing.

Lily set the pan of water on the little table, then pushed the door completely closed. She did everything required to tend Arabelle. It took some doing, but Lily rolled her onto her side so she could wash every part of her. And when she did so, she noticed a small bed sore on Arabelle's backside. Lily nearly asked if it hurt, but clamped her mouth shut remembering the poor woman didn't feel a thing.

"Arabelle . . ." Lily cleared her throat. "You have a sore that needs tendin'. Do you have medicine here in the house, or should I fix a poultice? I reckon I can find what it takes to make a good one."

"There's ointment in the top drawer of my bureau. Use that."

"So . . . you've had these before?"

She nodded, but said nothing.

Lily went to the bureau and found the medicine. "Would you like me to get my mirror, so you can see what the sore looks like? I have a hand-held mirror in my room. If you twist around just right, you can see what I'm talkin' 'bout."

"Heavens no. Why would I care to see such a thing?"

"Aren't you curious? If I had sumthin' like that, I'd wanna see it. An' since you can't *feel* it, I'd think you'd be even more interested. Don't you wanna know all that's goin' on with your body?"

Arabelle eyed her closely. "I know very well what's going on with my body. And I hate it." She leered at Lily. "You're an unusual girl. Now, doctor my wound and let me be."

"All right." Though utterly disheartened, Lily carefully dabbed medicine on the open sore. "You best lay on your side till this heals."

Arabelle voiced no comment. Lily decided to just push on and do her job. She dressed Arabelle in a clean nightgown. But even after freshening her clothes, the room still had a stale, unpleasant odor.

The bedding hadn't been soiled, but Lily was certain that at some time it must've been. "How long has it been since your beddin's been changed?"

"I don't recall."

"Then I'd say it's high time." Lily gulped. This wouldn't get easier anytime soon. "I'm gonna help you into your wheelchair, so I can change these sheets. The children are gatherin' up laundry. They said Mrs. Wood does it for y'all. When does she usually come?" She spoke fast, hoping to keep Arabelle from objecting.

"You have my children *working*?"

"They see it as a game." Lily pointed toward the door. "Can't you hear 'em laughin'? They're havin' a good time."

"Mrs. Wood picks up laundry every Wednesday and returns it on Friday." Arabelle made no remark about the children's laughter.

"Good. Then she'll be here t'morra. Reckon she'll have more to do than she bargained for." Lily let out a small laugh, but when Arabelle remained stone cold, she stifled it. "All right, then. Let me help you into the wheelchair."

Lily positioned it beside the bed. She placed a soft pillow on the hard seat. Of course, it wasn't meant for Arabelle's comfort, but rather as a means to help protect her delicate skin. Lily wanted to do all she could to prevent more lesions.

She situated herself next to Arabelle, then managed to get her arms around the woman and brought her to an upright position. Carefully, she scooted her to the edge of the bed.

Lily had never been more grateful for her strength. Though small-framed, Arabelle's dead weight was difficult to manage. Lily hoisted her up and landed her rather ungracefully into the chair.

Arabelle breathed hard. Her hands shook, and it looked as if she was trying to grasp the arms of the wheelchair, but her fingers barely moved.

"I'm sorry ma'am." Lily readjusted her in the seat. "We'll get better at this."

"I certainly hope so." Tears beaded up in Arabelle's eyes.

Lily found the handkerchief from the previous night and put it in her hand. "Here. I didn't mean to make you cry."

The small soft cloth drifted to the floor.

Lily picked it up and questioned Arabelle with her eyes.

"I don't have the strength to hold it." Arabelle's hands hadn't stopped trembling. "I can't do anything for myself. I thought you were aware of that."

Lily sat on the edge of her bed. "Your husband told me you're paralyzed from the waist down. I assumed you'd have full use of your arms an' hands."

"Well, I *don't*." She jerked her chin toward the bed. "Change it quickly, so I can lie down again."

"Yes'm." Lily stripped the bed faster than ever.

Arabelle directed her to the wardrobe, where Lily found more sheets. But what truly caught her eye were the abundance of beautiful gowns. Grown-up versions of the dresses the girls wore.

"Arabelle . . ." Lily glanced over her shoulder at the woman. "These are lovely. Want me to dress you in one?"

"No. What's the sense in that? I'll be lying down. A nightgown is the appropriate attire." She huffed a breath. "I'm cold. Hurry up with the sheets so you can put me in my bed."

"Yes'm." Lily grabbed the white linens and shut the wardrobe. In no time at all, she had the sheets smoothed over the bed and perfectly tucked in.

It was somewhat easier putting Arabelle back in the bed, than it had been getting her out of it. After positioning her on her side, Lily propped pillows behind her to keep her from rolling onto her wound, then she placed extra blankets over the top of her.

"Better?" Lily asked.

"Yes."

"Shall I bring you breakfast?"

"No. I'd like to sleep."

"But—"

"I said I'd like to sleep."

"Yes'm." Lily nearly turned to leave, yet something compelled her to stroke Arabelle's hair in a comforting gesture.

Her action brought a slim smile to the woman's face. She shut her eyes and burrowed deeper into the pillow beneath her head.

"I'll come back later," Lily whispered and left the room.

Because of Aunt Helen, Lily had grown accustomed to being around a short-tempered woman. But Arabelle was different. Hiding under her cold demeanor lay a loving soul. Of that, Lily had no doubt.

Arabelle was broken in many ways, and Lily intended to fix her.

* * *

"Father!" The girls raced to Mr. Jacobson's side. He'd barely gotten through the door.

Lily laughed and set Levi on the floor. The sweet boy toddled quickly to join the others.

Mr. Jacobson let out his own laugh. "What a wonderful greeting."

The girls all spoke at once, and not even Lily could make out what they were saying.

Mr. Jacobson held up a hand. "Slow down. One at a time. Oldest first." He nodded at Winnie.

"Father, we played a game today with the laundry, and I won!"

"She cheated," Jenny whined. "She took the things Levi gathered and claimed them as her own."

Winnie scowled. "I did not!"

"Did too!"

"Hush!" Opal fisted her hands on her hips. "Don't you remember what Miss Larsen said?"

Winnie and Jenny simultaneously looked Lily's way. "Sorry, Miss Larsen," they said in unison.

Levi tugged at his pa's pantleg. "I help."

Mr. Jacobson lifted him. "Good boy." He gazed beyond the children and took in the living room. "It's clean. I must say, Miss Larsen, you've worked hard today."

"We *all* did," Winnie said.

"That's right." Opal took her sister's hand. "Miss Larsen showed us what to do, and we did it. Don't the house look pretty?"

"*Doesn't*," Lily loudly whispered.

Opal swayed side to side. "*Doesn't* the house look pretty, Father?"

"Yes. Very pretty. But not as lovely as you three." He tapped the tip of each of their noses in turn.

Jenny's face screwed together. "But we're wearing ugly dresses."

He eyed them up and down. "I hadn't noticed. You look beautiful to me."

Levi rested his head against his pa's chest. The sight made Lily smile. Yes, he was a daddy's boy, but she'd won the boy over and hoped that tomorrow they'd have an easier start to their day.

Mr. Jacobson sniffed the air. "Something smells wonderful."

"Lily made vegetable soup," Opal said. "And muffins, too."

"Excellent." He set Levi down and removed his coat. Once he was free of it, the boy reached for him and was immediately picked up again.

"Why don't you children wash for supper?" Lily said. "You can tell your pa more 'bout what we did today while we eat."

"But Miss Larsen . . ." Winnie eyed her curiously. "We were taught not to speak with our mouths full."

"That's right." Lily cast her sternest *Mrs. Gottlieb* expression. "It's not appropriate. So, you chew, swallow, an' *then* talk." She grinned. "Now go wash."

They rushed to the wash basin and took turns.

Mr. Jacobson walked to the kitchen, his smile broader than ever. "I knew you'd do well, but I didn't expect all this."

"Don't be praisin' me too much. I didn't do quite so good with your wife."

"No? What happened?" He pulled out a chair and sat.

"She's stayed in bed all day. Wouldn't eat hardly anythin'. I hope *you* can get her to eat some soup."

"I'll see to it. She probably needs time to get used to you. It's not easy having someone else feed you."

Lily took a seat beside him and thrummed her fingers on the tabletop. She'd be taking a risk telling her employer how to treat his wife, but she couldn't remain silent. "She shouldn't *hafta* be fed. If she can strengthen her arms, she'll be able to do it herself."

"But how can she? She has no mobility."

"I can work with her. It'll take time, yet I know we can get her muscles strong again. She'll never walk, but she can do a lot with her hands."

No joy remained in his expression. "She used to tat. Made all the lovely lace for the girls' dresses."

"Then we should get her tattin' again." Lily scooted closer and lowered her voice. "Your wife needs purpose. She hasta see that she still has value."

"Of course she has value. She means the world to me."

Lily nodded. Her heart ached for the man. "I can tell you love her, but she's stopped lovin' herself. I wanna show her that her life's not over. She might get ill with me, but I hope you don't mind if I try."

He stared blankly at her and mindlessly rubbed Levi's back. The child's eyes were shut, and since he hadn't napped all day, Lily assumed he was truly asleep. "Want me to take Levi so you can go look in on Arabelle?"

He hesitated, shifting his eyes from the child to her. "I'm afraid he'll cry."

"Give me a chance. He an' I became friends today. I think he'll do just fine."

"All right." He tentatively passed the boy over and Levi cuddled against her.

He felt like a piece of heaven in her arms. "You see. No need for you to fret." She lifted her chin toward Arabelle's room. "Go on to your wife. I'm sure she'll tell you 'bout the wheelchair."

"What about it?" Mr. Jacobson stood.

"Let *her* tell you. An' think 'bout what I said. I truly believe I can help her regain her strength."

"All right. I'll give it some thought."

He wandered away to the bedroom and shut the door.

Lily gathered the children together. She shifted sleepy Levi onto her shoulder, and held him while the girls set the table. The boy seemed small for his age. Perhaps he'd taken after his ma rather than his pa. But if Lily was recalling Isaac and Horace correctly, they were quite a bit larger than Levi when they'd turned two.

She couldn't deny she enjoyed every second she spent with the child in her arms. Having him so small made him easier to hold.

Winnie set the final plate on the table. "We should wait for Father before we sit down to eat."

Lily smiled at her. "That's very kind. I'm sure he'll appreciate it."

When he finally came out of the bedroom, his head hung low.

Winnie hurried to his side. "What's wrong, Father?"

"Your mother is miserable." He took a large breath and stared at Lily. "Do whatever you can to help her."

Lily smiled and nodded, but inwardly she shouted with gratitude.

Tomorrow, there'd be more games to play.

If all went as she hoped, they'd have an additional player.

Chapter 10

Lily woke to the same clinking sound she'd heard the day before. One thing was certain. Mr. Jacobson had a routine.

The positive attitude she'd seen coming from him the moment they'd met had briefly vanished last night. She assumed he buried many of his feelings deep inside. From what she'd learned of men, they often liked to appear strong for their families, while they suffered inwardly.

If she could help his wife, it would help him, too.

She flipped her covers off and hopped out of bed. Having a purpose sure helped *her* attitude.

Her brown dress lay where she'd left it. She studied it for a mere second, then put on her blue one. Though fancier than she liked for the kind of work she had to do, the other dress needed to be laundered. And since they expected Mrs. Wood today, it wouldn't hurt to add her dirty brown dress to the large pile.

She quickly fixed her hair, then headed to the kitchen.

Levi obviously had a routine as well. He sat cuddled against his pa. When the boy caught sight of her, he grinned. Lily wiggled her fingers at him, casting her own smile.

Mr. Jacobson lifted his head, then pointed to the pot of coffee.

She poured herself a cup and took a seat beside him. "It's another lovely day." She gazed toward the kitchen window. "I thought I'd take the children outside for a while. Maybe work the garden a bit."

He slowly nodded. "What are your plans for my wife?"

"I'd love to get *her* outside, too. She could use some sunshine an' fresh air."

His shoulders dropped. "I've tried. She refuses. It bothers her to think that people might see her in that chair." He grunted. "As if anyone would be troubled by it. Everyone in the city knows about her condition."

"You're right. No one would think anythin' of seein' her that way. But *she's* embarrassed. She doesn't like seein' *herself* disabled."

His head drew back. "How'd you get so wise?"

Lily took a sip of her drink. Mrs. Gottlieb would be proud of her right now. "I learned a lot from my pa. He lost an arm in the war. For months, he wallowed in self-pity. Drank too much. Let our farm go by the wayside. I had to keep the family goin'. Then someone came into our lives who showed him his capabilities. Got him to see that his life still had meanin'. This person didn't go easy on my pa, but that's what he needed. Someone to be firm, but caring."

"How's your father doing now?"

"I reckon he's fine. I haven't heard from my folks in a great while. But my sister tells me that the farm's doin' well. Pa had to hire extra hands to tend it."

Mr. Jacobson cradled his cup of coffee. "That's good. And what of the person who helped him? Is he still there?"

"How'd you know it was a he?"

The man shrugged. "If your father was in such poor condition and a woman as strong as yourself couldn't bring him out of his slump, then I assumed it took a *very* strong man."

"It did. An' no, he's not there now. He went home." She turned away. Her throat dried and her chest constricted. If they didn't talk about something else, she'd likely cry.

A soft touch sent chills along her arm. When she looked at it, Levi's tiny hand rested there.

Oh, my . . .

Had the dear child sensed her pain?

She took a deep breath to push down tears, then grabbed hold of his hand and kissed it. "You're such a sweet boy."

He stretched his arms out to her.

Mr. Jacobson's eyes widened, but Lily didn't hesitate taking the boy. She cuddled him close and breathed him in. Simply holding him soothed her and kept her from crying.

"Well . . ." Mr. Jacobson set his coffee on the table and folded his arms over his chest. "You've definitely made a difference to my son."

Lily gently swayed with the child. "I love holdin' him, but his ma should be doin' this. He needs her."

"You're right." He released a long sigh. "If you're able to build her strength, then maybe she can hold him." He scooted his chair back and got to his feet.

Lily remained seated with Levi resting against her.

Mr. Jacobson walked across the room and headed to the front door. He paused and glanced back at them, then grabbed his coat.

When he opened the door, he hesitated once again. She understood why. He'd expected Levi to come after him, crying. But the boy didn't budge. Lily saw it as a step forward, but the child's behavior probably hurt his pa a mite.

Mr. Jacobson dipped his head. "I hope you have a successful day." He disappeared out the door.

Levi lifted his head. "Papa work."

"Yes, he hasta work. An' now it's our turn. Shall we get your sisters outta bed?"

He giggled and squirmed from her lap. The next thing she knew, he was shuffling across the floor to the girls' bedroom.

Grinning, Lily got to her feet and followed.

* * *

Once breakfast was over, Levi seemed content on the floor with a stack of building blocks, and Lily got the girls busy cleaning and straightening their rooms. Of course, they teased her about her fancy blue dress, but had no problem putting on their *ugly* dresses—as they'd come to call them.

She promised to take the children outside once the interior of the house was in order, and had even mentioned the possibility of carving a pumpkin for Halloween.

Their excited chatter filled the house, but as before, Lily knew that the most difficult tasks lay ahead of her, and they had nothing to do with the children.

She approached Arabelle as she had previously. The woman never called out to her, but Lily went into her room and found her wide awake. Lily took it upon herself to change her, without even asking permission. They had to establish a routine, and this seemed to be the way to start it.

Arabelle kept her eyes shifted from Lily. "There's no need to put me in the wheelchair today. My bedding is fine."

"Yes, it is." Lily made certain Arabelle was completely clean and dry before doctoring her wound. It appeared to be slightly better already. "I'd like to do sumthin' else today."

"What might that be?"

"I noticed your brush on the bureau. May I tend your hair?" Lily prayed for a *yes*. She herself loved having someone else groom her hair. It always relaxed her. After the way Arabelle had responded to Lily's touch last night, she believed Arabelle felt the same.

Finally, the woman looked at her. "I suppose you may. As long as you take care with the tangles. I still have plenty of feeling in my head."

"An' that's a very good thing." Lily smiled and grabbed the brush. She perched on the edge of the bed, then helped Arabelle into an upright position. "Are you comfortable?"

"I'm a little chilled."

Lily got up and repositioned the blankets high around Arabelle's body. "Better?"

"Yes. Thank you."

"You're welcome." She sat again and lifted the brush. "Your hair could use a good washin'." She gently drew the brush through a long strand. "Perhaps we'll tackle that t'morra."

"Perhaps."

Lily continued on. She occasionally ran into a mass of tangles, but worked with them until they smoothed out. She'd learned how to manage unruly hair by helping Violet with hers. "I noticed some fine hats in your wardrobe. Maybe someday, we'll go into town an' you can wear one."

Arabelle scowled. "I won't go into town. Get those silly notions out of your head."

"All right." Lily kept on brushing until Arabelle's hair was completely smooth and shiny, then she lowered the brush and faced her directly. "Will you do sumthin' for me?"

"That depends on what it is."

Lily took hold of her hands. "I want you to squeeze as hard as you can."

"I told you, I can't. I have no strength."

"Prove it."

Arabelle's eyes narrowed, then her dainty hands trembled, and her fingers lightly curled around Lily's.

It gave her hope. "That's good, Arabelle."

"How can it be good? I applied no pressure at all."

"But you moved your fingers. That's a start." Lily set the brush within Arabelle's reach. "I'm gonna leave this here. You should practice squeezin' it as often as you can. Will you do that for me?"

"Why?"

"Your husband told me you used to tat. The work you did on the girls' dresses is beautiful. Wouldn't you like to do it again?"

Arabelle frowned, but her head slightly lifted. "How could I?"

"Your arms an' hands aren't paralyzed, they just need to remember what it's like to be used. I *know* we can get them workin' again."

Arabelle gradually moved her right hand under the brush and her fingers slowly circled it. Her lips rose into a smile.

Lily's heart leapt. "I made some biscuits an' gravy for breakfast. Are you hungry?"

"Yes. I think I am. But—"

"Don't fret, Arabelle. For now, I can feed you. In time, I know you'll be able to do it yourself." Lily cast an encouraging smile and left her to ponder what she'd said.

The fact Arabelle had an appetite was already a great improvement over the previous day.

* * *

It pleased Lily to see Arabelle eat as much as she had, and now the woman was resting. Something she was very good at. Still, they'd made progress.

Lily shut the door to her bedroom and nearly tumbled over Opal.

The girl tugged on Lily's arm. "Can we get the pumpkin now?"

"All right. But you've gotta get your shoes on."

The children wasted no time. Lily helped Levi into his shoes, then she made sure everyone bundled up in a coat.

The crisp October air greeted them. Truthfully, it felt wonderful. Lily inhaled the scent of fall and gazed toward the mountains. *Her* mountains.

Home.

Levi stretched his arms upward and wiggled his fingers. She scooped him from the ground and headed for the weedy garden.

The girls chatter followed them. Giggles mixed with a small amount of whining. Not surprising at all, Jenny didn't care for the cold.

Winnie pointed at the mass of tangled weeds and grass. "I see a big pumpkin in there."

"Me, too." Jenny squatted next to the garden. "Right there." She extended a stiff finger. "But it's dirty."

Lily laughed and set Levi down. "Course it is. But I think it's ready to be picked. In fact . . ." She pushed aside a mass of dry grass. "I reckon we can find a pumpkin for each of you."

Opal's eyes popped wide. "I get my own?"

"Yep."

Levi plopped onto his rump beside his sister. "Me, too." He patted the hard ground, then rubbed his bottom. "Cold."

"Yes, it is." Every time she looked at the boy, love overwhelmed her. He was too cute for his own good. "I want each of you to find a pumpkin you like. Then we'll take 'em inside, clean 'em up, an' decide how we're gonna carve 'em."

Jenny fisted her hands on her hips. "How do you know how to do that?"

Lily's memories rushed in like a flash flood. "Before the war came an' changed how we lived, folks in the cove would gather every year on the final Saturday of October for a fall festival. Each family would bring a carved pumpkin, an' everyone would vote for their favorite. My family never won, but I learned how to skillfully use a knife to create a decent face. Or at least one my brothers could laugh at."

Opal giggled.

"So, what would you like?" Lily asked. "Do you want your pumpkin silly or scary?"

"Scary," Winnie said.

Opal splayed her arms wide. "Silly, of course."

Jenny screwed her mouth together, then tipped her head to the side. "Can mine look like a fairy princess?"

"We'll see." The girls definitely had unique personalities. Lily patted Levi's head. "What do you want yours to be?"

"Papa."

Opal giggled louder. "Maybe we can put glasses on Levi's pumpkin and give it a big nose. Then it'll look like Father."

Levi rapidly nodded.

It took some doing, but Lily managed to entice the girls into getting their hands dirty. Even Jenny. The garden needed a lot of work, but for now, they'd enjoy the pumpkins and make a special holiday memory. Lily could add it to her many others.

She found a few squashes that were also ready to be picked. They'd be delicious with supper.

They cleaned the pumpkins, then put them on the kitchen table. Lily found a knife suitable for the task at hand. "This is sharp, so I'll do the cuttin', but you can guide me how you want it. First, we hafta get the guts out."

Jenny's nose wrinkled. "Guts?"

"Yep." Lily put a pan on the table, then carefully cut the tops off each pumpkin. She took a large spoon and dug into the first one, scooping out the slimy pulp and seeds.

"Yuck!" Opal also scrunched up her face. "That's icky."

The children peered at the mess, making the sourest faces ever.

Lily kept scooping. "You haven't done this before, have you?"

"Uh-uh," Winnie said. "We've only seen jack-o-lanterns at parties. Mother and Father took Jenny and me when we were little. But we haven't been to a Halloween party in a long time. We didn't know pumpkins had guts."

"Have you ever eaten the seeds?"

"No. Are they good?"

Lily grinned. "*Very* good. But we have to separate 'em from the *guts*, then clean 'em an' roast 'em. Who wants to pull the seeds out of the guts?"

Jenny backed away from the table.

Winnie stood tall. "I will."

"Good girl." Lily gestured to an empty pot. "You'll hafta get your hands in the stuff I scooped out, then pull out the seeds an' put them in that pot."

Winnie dug right in. "It's gooey." She squinted her eyes, but kept going.

Levi wiggled in next to her. "I help."

Before Lily could stop him, he was up to his elbows in goo. No seeds went into the pan from his tiny hands, but plenty of orange pulp got stuck in his hair.

They had a lot of laughs, followed by baths. And since all the pumpkins were done and the children were nice and clean, the time had come for Lily to take one last step.

The children proudly held their carved pieces. Winnie's had fangs and large wide eyes. Opals was cross-eyed and had its tongue sticking out. Jenny adorned hers with a toy tiara she brought from her room, and Lily made sure it had long, girlish eyelashes and pretty, nicely formed lips. As for Levi, they managed to find an old pair of his pa's glasses to put on his pumpkin. Lily gave it a fitting broad smile and a large nose—hoping Mr. Jacobson had a good sense of humor—and cut little holes in the side of it to place the eyewear, so the glasses wouldn't slip off.

Lily stepped back and admired their work. "We should show these to your ma."

"But . . ." Winnie frowned. "She's sleeping."

"No, I'm not."

Every head whipped around and faced Arabelle's bedroom. Her voice had come through clearly.

Had she been listening all this time?

Though Lily was more than surprised, she chose to hide it. It was important for the children to know their ma wanted to be with them.

"All right, then," she said. "Let's go in an' show your ma what you've done." She led them across the floor like a parade, pushed Arabelle's door wide open, and marched them inside.

They stood beside her bed in a perfect row.

Lily hurried to Arabelle and helped her sit up. Her hair had retained its nicely brushed finish. She looked lovely.

"I need more light," Arabelle said. "Can you open the drapes?"

"Gladly." Lily pushed them all the way back and let the sunshine stream in.

"Look at what you've done." Arabelle choked out the words. "They're wonderful."

Levi climbed atop the bed, toting his *pa*. Luckily, it was the smallest pumpkin in the patch and he capably handled it.

He set the thing on his ma's legs. "It's Papa."

"I can see that." Arabelle's chin quivered and she teared up.

"Don't cry, Mother." Winnie moved closer. "We didn't mean to make you sad."

"I'm not." She swallowed so hard, Lily heard it. "I'm proud of you. All of you." Her eyes lifted to Lily's, and she smiled. "Thank you."

Lily dipped her head. "Tell you what. I'm gonna go get the pumpkin seeds ready to roast. I'll let the children entertain you for a spell. They can tell you all 'bout their pumpkins an' why they chose to have me make the faces the way I did."

She eased out of the room to the sound of overly excited children. Their love for their ma was evident, but Lily never doubted it for a minute.

More importantly, she knew Arabelle felt the same. But she'd been so caught up in her own misery, she'd forgotten what it was like to be their mother. They needed her and she needed them.

No one knew that better than Lily.

Tonight, she'd write letters. She had to know that Noah was well. And maybe it was time to reconcile with her own ma. She'd write to her with all the good memories in mind from her childhood, and cast aside the recollection of the pain her folks had caused by making her leave and taking Noah from her.

Somehow, they all had to heal.

Chapter 11

All the excitement of having the children in her room seemed to have worn Arabelle down, so Lily shuffled them out to let their ma sleep. They chatted nonstop and hovered around her as if waiting for her to take them on another adventure. Honestly, Lily couldn't recall when she'd enjoyed carving pumpkins so much.

While Arabelle napped, Lily put Levi down for his own long rest. The boy didn't fuss about being put to bed. His head hit the pillow, and his eyes shut.

Plumb tuckered out.

Lily stared at his sleeping form for a few moments, but the girls' impatient voices were growing louder, and Lily didn't want them to wake Levi or his ma. Perhaps teaching the girls how to bake biscuits would simmer them down.

It amazed Lily that they'd never been exposed to such things. From all they'd told her, everything they needed was provided to them from one source or another. Their pa bartered for everyday essentials. Being the owner of a store certainly helped his leverage.

They got their eggs from a woman named Mrs. Dent, milk and butter from Mr. Armstrong, and baked goods—like bread and such—from Mrs. Tomlinson. According to Winnie, they'd been acquiring their goods that way since before their ma had been hurt. And of course, Mrs. Wood took care of all their laundry.

No wonder Arabelle had had the time to make lace and keep a clean house. She'd had little else to do. Lily couldn't imagine being so pampered.

The door opened unexpectedly, and Lily jumped.

Opal let out one of her precious giggles. "It's Father!"

The girls raced to greet him, and like before, each talked at the same time. Levi even joined in, babbling something undiscernible. He hadn't slept as long as Lily had thought he would. He'd woken as soon as the scent of baking biscuits hit the air.

It amazed Lily how quickly the afternoon had flown by. She wiped her hands on her apron and hurried across the room to join the chaos. "We've had quite the day."

The man chuckled. "I'm trying to get details, but it's nearly impossible." He pointed over his shoulder. "I passed Mrs. Wood on the road. The back of her wagon is nearly full of laundry. That wasn't all ours, was it?"

"'Fraid so," Lily said. "The children hunted high an' low an' found all kinds a dirty things. Next week shouldn't be so bad."

"No wonder she had such a large smile when I passed her. I'll owe her a great deal in goods." His smile broadened. "Don't misunderstand me. I'm thankful I can help her." His expression sobered. "How's Arabelle?"

"She talked to us today," Winnie said, wide-eyed, before Lily could answer. "*All* of us."

A shame that such a simple act was seen as an accomplishment, but Lily fully understood. She, too, was pleased with how the day had gone.

Mr. Jacobson's expression brightened once again. He moved beside Lily and peered into her eyes. "So, her mood has improved?"

"Yes. The children spent a great while with her, showin' her the pumpkins we carved. That is—*I* carved. I'd never let a child handle a knife that way. They told me how they wanted them to look, then I cut out the features. You should go an' see them for yourself. They're lined up on your bureau."

Opal tugged at his coat sleeve. "Miss Larsen says we'll put candles in them and light them at night. Won't that be lovely?"

He lifted her into his arms. "Yes, it will." He tickled under her chin and prompted more giggles. Maybe that's where they'd truly began. Since she'd been the baby of the family for a number of years before Levi had come along, Lily assumed she'd been a daddy's girl, too.

Lily took in the faces of all the children and in a very different way became tickled herself. Levi eyed Opal as if to say, *you don't belong there, I do.*

Opal wrapped her arms around her pa's neck and hugged him. Once that happened, Levi turned his attention to Lily. He rushed to her and reached upward. "Hold me."

Lily scooped the jealous child from the floor. "Don't worry, Levi," she whispered in his ear. "Your pa has plenty a love for all of you." She kissed his cheek.

Mr. Jacobson returned Opal to the floor. "I'll make certain Arabelle's awake, then we can all go in and see the pumpkins together." He nodded at Lily. "You, too."

It didn't take long for him to call them into the room. He waved a hand out the door and gestured for them to enter. His smile reached his ears.

Lily stood back and watched the family interact. Joy filled the space as the children shared their stories.

Fortunately, Mr. Jacobson laughed at his jack-o-lantern image. He bent low and peered into the carved face. "I don't believe justice was done to my nose. It's not quite *large* enough." He looked over his shoulder and grinned at Lily.

She smiled back at him, then moved her attention to Arabelle. He'd propped her up on the pillows, and she appeared to be fairly comfortable. Lily noticed the hairbrush close to her hand.

"Arthur?" Arabelle's voice sounded quite different addressing him. Softer and not so demanding. "I'd like to show you what I did today."

The room fell silent.

Mr. Jacobson knelt beside the bed. "Yes, dear?"

She looked at the hairbrush, and drew his eyes to it.

Lily held her breath.

Arabelle's hand crept so slowly, it felt as if time had stopped. She inched it under the ceramic brush. Her fingers quivered. A large muscle spasm rapidly jerked her hand, and the brush fell to the floor.

No . . .

Arabelle gasped. "I can't do it!" She leered at Lily. "You shouldn't have made me try."

Mr. Jacobson gave Lily his own look—one of confusion. "What was she supposed to do?"

Every eye in the room rested on Lily. She wasn't about to be defeated. The day had been too glorious.

She bent down and retrieved the hairbrush, then moved next to Arabelle. "Try again. Your muscles hafta remember what to do."

Arabelle shook her head. "It's no use."

"Children," Mr. Jacobson sternly said. "Leave the room."

No. It couldn't end this way. Lily chose to be bold. "Wait. I want them to see what I *know* she can do."

All four small faces turned to their pa.

He breathed deeply, then held up a hand. "Fine. They may stay. But try not to further upset my wife."

Lily jutted her chin and set the brush within Arabelle's reach. "Go ahead. It'll be fine this time."

Arabelle shut her eyes, then reopened them and glided her hand once again beneath the hairbrush. Perhaps she'd said a prayer, or maybe she was building up courage. Whatever the reason for closing her eyes, Lily believed that had she not been there, Arabelle may never have done another thing but lie in bed. *Forever.* Her husband was too soft on her to challenge her to do more.

Arabelle's fingers curled around the brush. She squinted and tightened them even more. "I'm doing it!"

The girls cheered and Mr. Jacobson simply stood there, gaping. Levi clapped his hands and laughed, but Lily doubted he understood his ma's accomplishment.

"You see, Arthur." Arabelle hadn't let go of the brush. "My hands have to remember what to do. Lily said I'll get stronger, but I have to work at it."

Mr. Jacobson kissed her forehead. "I'm so proud of you." They locked eyes.

Lily recognized that expression. "Children, your folks need to talk some alone. Let's go finish up supper."

They took turns hugging their ma, then followed Lily to the kitchen.

She gestured to the table. "I wanna talk 'bout what just happened, so everyone sit."

The girls obeyed without question. Once Lily was seated, Levi climbed onto her lap.

"Your ma," Lily said, "is gonna hafta practice real hard to get her hands workin' again. See, it takes muscles to move our bodies. Hers have gotten soft an' weak."

"Is that why she don't hug too good?" Opal asked.

"Yes. That's why she *doesn't* hug very well." Lily smiled at the child. "But we can all help her by movin' her arms for her an' rubbin' them real good to get her blood pumpin'. I know it'd help her legs, too."

"But she can't feel anything in her legs," Winnie said. "Why should we rub *them*?"

"Cuz our bodies were made to move." Lily didn't know quite how to explain it. "All I know is—if blood doesn't get to every inch a your body, that part a you will die."

Jenny's eyes popped wide. "We don't want mother to *die*."

"No. No. No." Lily waved her hands. "That's not what I meant. Your ma is healthy. But since her legs can't feel nothin', they're kinda sick. She can't make 'em strong on her own, so we gotta help. Understand?"

Jenny shifted her mouth from side to side. "I suppose." She sat a bit taller. "Can I dress her up? I can take the tiara off my pumpkin and put it on *her*."

"In time, we can fix her up in some a the hats she already has." Lily leaned in and lowered her voice. "But we gotta take this slow. One step at a time. Muscles now, hats later. All right?"

Every head bobbed.

"Good. T'morra you'll all help me with her. I know she loves havin' you close. Give her lotsa hugs an' smiles, an' soon, she'll be the ma you remember."

Winnie frowned and shook her head. "But she can't walk."

"That doesn't matter. It's her heart that counts the most, an' all she needs is your love. When she accepts the wheelchair, she'll be able to walk in her own way."

Levi cuddled closer. "I hungry."

"Reckon it's time to eat. But you'll hafta let me get up."

He shook his head and held on tighter.

Lily laughed. "Silly boy."

Winnie stood and came to her side. "C'mon, Levi. Let Miss Larsen cook. If you don't, none of us will eat." She extended her hand.

Levi eyed it for a second, then took it and wiggled off Lily's lap and onto the floor.

The girls set about preparing the table for the meal, while Lily put the final touches on supper. In only a few short days, she'd become a part of this family and their daily routine. But something struck her that she hadn't considered before.

She turned to the two oldest girls. "Y'all seem to know a great deal. Is there a school you attend?"

Jenny sighed. "No schools. Our mother used to teach us. Winnie and I know all our letters and are good spellers. We also know how to work numbers. But Opal and Levi won't know anything, unless *you* teach them."

It seemed Lily had something else to add to her long list of to-dos. Then again, she'd uncovered something more that Arabelle could capably do right away. Teaching the children didn't require the movement of her legs or even her hands for that matter.

"Hmm . . ."

Lily had a lot to ponder.

Chapter 12

It took Violet more than a few days to calm down enough to venture back to her folks' cabin. And when they were absent from Sunday services, it made things even worse. Normally, Violet was able to get at least a peek at Noah on Sundays.

"Stardust . . ." She patted the mare's side. "I reckon Ma purposefully stayed home from church to keep me from seein' Noah."

The horse kept plodding along and gave no reaction to her remark. Why she expected one, had her even more concerned about herself.

"Maybe Gideon was right when he called me crazy." She sat high in the saddle, taking her time on the road. "Course, that was 'fore we were married, an' he was wrong, but . . ."

She shook her head.

Stop talkin' to the horse.

What she really should be thinking about was what to say to her pa. She'd made up her mind to see him, but feared she'd ramble on and say something inappropriate and make him angry.

A cool breeze dusted her face. She shivered, wishing she'd put on another layer of clothes. November approached. Soon after, they'd have snow. She loved the exquisiteness of the white blanket that covered the endless fields and the icy crystals that clung to every tree branch. Yet, she hated the cold.

November.

Last November she'd witnessed a miracle. At the time, she'd seen it as disturbing—something her ma had forced her to watch. Thinking back on it now, it had been a beautiful thing. Her sweet nephew had come into the world.

Then everything changed.

If she thought about it too hard, she'd get angry again and might be hateful to her pa. He didn't deserve that from her. Maybe he wasn't aware how badly she wanted to see Noah.

She needed to give the man the benefit of the doubt.

Her poor nose was icy cold, so she cupped a hand over her face and breathed out a nice, warm breath. It helped for a few seconds, then it seemed even colder.

What she truly wished for was her backside in front of a roaring fire. That, or her husband's arms around her.

The thought alone helped to heat her. Gideon had been extra loving since she'd been so ill about the situation with Noah. The man was more considerate of her than she felt she deserved most of the time. No husband could be better.

Those happy thoughts led her to her folks' place, but as she neared it, some of her ugly feelings returned.

She didn't plan to stay long, so she tied Stardust to a tree and marched up the steps to the cabin. The door opened before she even knocked.

"Violet?" Her ma's sour face greeted her. "You sound like a herd a elk on the porch. What are you doin' stompin' like that, an' why are you here?"

She'd stay calm for Noah's sake. "I came to visit. I was worried when you weren't in church on Sunday." She peered beyond her ma into the cabin.

"Well, get inside 'fore you let the warm air out." Her ma stepped back and opened the door just enough for Violet to squeeze through.

Isaac raced to her side. "Did you come to play charades like we used to?"

"No, I'm afraid not." His face fell, so she bent to his level. "Least not right now. I wanna talk to pa first. All right?"

"I s'pose." He kicked at the floor.

Horace lifted his head from the sofa and cast a slim smile, then returned to a picture he was drawing on his slate.

The crackling fire beckoned Violet, but concern over Noah took precedence. He wasn't to be seen.

"What do you want Pa for?" Isaac asked.

Her ma came close. "I was wonderin' that very thing."

Violet's mind spun. She hadn't thought this part through. "Well . . . Christmas is comin'. It's 'bout a Christmas surprise, so I can't say no more." It seemed reasonable enough. Christmastime always held secrets.

"Hmm." Her ma scowled and waved a hand. "Ain't gonna be much of a Christmas this year. Reckon them new relations a yours have more money than we do, an' can afford fancy gifts."

Violet gulped and bit her tongue, choosing to keep her mouth shut.

Her ma pointed outside. "Your pa's in the barn lookin' in on the livestock."

Violet feared what she needed to ask, expecting another glare. "An' . . . Noah?" She held her breath.

"He's nappin'." Her ma jerked her head toward the bedroom. The one Violet used to occupy with Lily. It had become Noah's room. The other two boys still slept in the loft.

Though relieved he was there, she had no excuse to go to him. Especially after saying she'd come to talk to her pa. Regardless, she wasted no time and strode across the room. The door was ajar, so she peeked in.

Her ma hadn't lied. Noah's small frame was huddled beneath a mound of blankets. They rose and fell with every breath he took.

She let out a relieved sigh, spun on her heels, and headed for the front door.

"Satisfied?" Her ma murmured.

Violet decided it wasn't worth responding to and walked out.

At least she could tell Lily that Noah was alive and well. But not a lot more than that considering her limited accessibility to the boy. The whole situation was ridiculous, but more than anything, infuriating.

She hugged her winter coat closer to her body and hurried to the barn.

Knowing her pa was alone, worked in her favor.

When the weather turned cold like this, he kept the doors to the barn shut to hold in as much heat as possible.

She eased inside and welcomed the scant amount of warmth and the scent of the animals. Though some of the odors were unpleasant, nasty smells meant prosperity. It hadn't been long ago that they had nothing but a few chickens. Most folks would look at her pa and think they were poor, but Violet knew better. Full bellies, enough wood to make a warm fire, and a place to lay their heads at night made them rich. Cove folks didn't require anything more than that to survive.

Violet's new family felt the same. However, they had something more that made each day gratifying. *Joyful* spirit. The Larsen home once had it, but it had gotten lost somewhere. Isaac retained some of it, but she'd seen it dwindle in Horace. Her ma's joy had vanished right after the war started. Violet had found hers again the day Gideon came back into her life.

Her pa was on the fence with his happiness. His happy spark had greatly dimmed after he'd sent Lily away, but Violet had seen some of it reignite the day of her wedding. Something she was grateful for.

"Pa?" She crept across the floor. A small part of her feared he'd returned to his old ways and she'd find him tipping the jug again.

She eyed the old hidden room. "Pa?"

The door creaked open and he stepped through. "Violet? I didn't expect you, but it's always good to see ya." He glanced back at where he'd come from, then faced her again.

Violet worked her lower lip. At least he hadn't slurred his words. "You all right, Pa?"

"Me?" He pointed to himself. "You don't think . . . Violet. I ain't got no moonshine. I keep some jerky in there an' nibble on it when Rose don't cook fast enough for my likin'." He grinned. "A man's gotta eat."

She ran to him and hugged him. "Sorry, Pa. But when you came out . . . I mean . . . well, you know."

"Yep, I do." He patted her back. "What brings you here?"

She stepped away from him and focused on the straw scattered across the floor. "I reckon I should just spit it out. Right?"

"Sounds serious. Sumthin' wrong at home?" He grabbed hold of her arm. "That husband a yours treatin' you proper?"

"Course he is." She looked him in the eyes. "Gideon's the kindest, most wonderful man I've ever known."

Her pa's head jerked back. "Better than your old pa?"

"Oh, Pa." She patted his lone arm. "You know you're special to me. But with Gideon, it's different."

"Yep. I understand. I'm just foolin' with ya." He pointed at a bale of straw. "Let's sit, so you can tell me what's on your mind."

She gladly sat. She pressed her body against one of the warmest men on earth and the straw shielded her backside from the cold. "It's Noah. I'm worried 'bout him."

Her pa's brows dipped low. "He sick or sumthin'? Your ma didn't say nothin' to me 'fore I came out here."

"No. He ain't sick, but . . ." She twisted her fingers together, then shifted on the bale and faced him. "Why did Ma hafta take him to the Henderson's? If she can't tend him, *I* wanna do it."

"That's what this is 'bout? You got sumthin' against Mrs. Henderson?"

"No." Violet rubbed her temples. "She's a fine woman. But she ain't kin. I don't understand why Ma has trouble keepin' Noah here with her. He's a good baby an' doesn't get into things. When I was here the other day, we was just peelin' apples. Noah coulda been there, sittin' on the floor at our feet, playin' or sumthin'. Why'd she hafta send him elsewhere?"

He took hold of her hand and cradled it in his large palm. "I'm gonna speak plain to you, Violet, cuz you're a grown woman an' should understand these kinda things. See—your ma ain't been right for some time now. I know you've seen how short-tempered an' ill she's gotten. An'—don't get me wrong—I love 'er, but she ain't the woman I married. I don't fully understand what happened to her.

"I figgered, once the war was over, she'd get back to bein' herself. But it's gotten worse. Not only can she be mean as a snake, she forgets things. Where she puts her belongin's an' such. The other day, I had to help her find the clothespins. They was right where she always left 'em, but she said they was missin'."

Violet listened intently to every word. She certainly hadn't expected this. "That makes no sense, Pa."

"No, it don't. An' this past Sunday we didn't go to church cuz Rose insisted it was Saturday. Then later in the day, when it was too late, she fussed at me for not takin' her to services. As for Noah, I don't worry so much when he's with the Hendersons. I can't keep my eye on the boy when I'm out here workin', an' I fear Rose might forget about him an' let him wander off."

Violet tightened her hold on his hand. "Then why not let *me* take him? You know I'd be good to 'im."

Her pa released her and cupped his hand to her face. "I know. But I agree with your ma on this one thing. We can't have you confusin' the boy into thinkin' *you're* his ma. Folks might start talkin'. They could say some ugly things 'bout our family."

Anger coursed through her, but she kept her voice calm. "Why's it always hafta be 'bout our good family name? A name ain't worth salt if the people bearin' it are empty inside. Horace rarely smiles anymore, an' Ma *never* does. If there's sumthin' wrong with her mind, maybe she should see a doctor. As for you—you put on a good front, but I know you miss Lily." The instant Violet said her name, tears bubbled up. "Don't tell me you don't. Ain't you worried 'bout where she is?"

He turned his head and put his back to her. Within seconds, his shoulders jerked and he started to cry. "Course I am. But there ain't nothin' I can do 'bout it. An' yes, I miss her every day."

"Have you ever thought a makin' this right? Give Noah back to her an' let her raise him. He needs a good ma. Not Mrs. Henderson!"

He spun around on the bale and sat tall. "I can't. We don't know where she is, an' even if we did, we couldn't give him back. If we told folks she was his ma, we'd be shunned by everyone here. No one would trust a thing we had to say. How could we live like that?"

Violet sucked in a rasping breath. "Seems to me you ain't livin' well now. An' the only reason *I'm* happy is cuz I *don't* live here. The Myers took me in as one a their own. Not only does Gideon love me, but they do, too. They're kind an' givin'. An'—"

"Go home, Violet." Her pa stood and walked over to one of the horse stalls. He braced his hand on the rail. "Go where you're happy, an' don't fret 'bout us. We'll be fine."

She clutched a hand to her heart, knowing she'd hurt him. "An' Noah?"

His eyes narrowed. "I won't let nothin' bad happen to *my* son. I love that boy. Don't never question that. Hear me?"

She swallowed the stone in her throat. "Yessir."

"I love you, too, Violet. An' your sister. But things gotta be this way. We dug ourselves in, an' there ain't no comin' out."

She couldn't utter another sound. Her heart ached too much.

She sped from the barn and mounted Stardust. Had she not promised Gideon that she wouldn't ride fast, she would've raced home. But she wouldn't break her word. Truth and honesty meant more to her now than ever before, and she was determined to keep her new family moral. Even if it meant letting go of the old one.

Chapter 13

Lily couldn't budge from her bed. Grief weighed her down. How could she face the day with a smile, when she wanted to do nothing more than sob and feel sorry for herself?

The Jacobsons weren't the problem. Her relationship with them had progressed better and faster than she'd ever expected. Not only did the children willingly help with chores whenever Lily asked, their folks didn't fuss at her for giving the girls so many responsibilities. Quite the opposite. They praised both her and their children for tasks well done.

The girls had also been assisting with Arabelle, taking turns rubbing her arms and legs. Levi added his own special abilities, which Lily believed were just as important as the work his sisters were doing. Maybe even more so. His time with his ma was spent laying by her side, cuddling against her shoulder. Physical contact they both required. Arabelle would often read to him, and her hands had gotten strong enough to stroke his tiny head.

His tiny head.

Lily burst into tears, flipped onto her stomach, and buried her face in the pillow.

"Miss Larsen?" Mr. Jacobson's muffled voice came through the shut door. He rapped lightly, but didn't enter.

Lily lifted her head and sucked in air. "I don't feel well."

No response.

She hoped he'd heard.

The door opened less than an inch. "Shall I get a doctor?"

"No." She tried to keep her words calm. "My stomach is upset. That's all. I'm sure it'll pass."

A soft murmur came from behind the man. He pushed the door a little wider. "Winnie said she can tend to her mother's changing, and she'll also see to breakfast. You should stay in bed and rest a while longer."

"Thank you." Why Winnie had gotten up so early troubled Lily. Maybe the entire household had heard her crying.

Mr. Jacobson shut the door, and Lily let her tears flow freely.

November the tenth. An entire year had passed since she'd given birth to her son.

I should be celebratin' with him, not cryin' over his loss.

She doubted her folks would do much of anything to honor the day. She'd written to them and Violet almost two weeks ago and prayed for a response sometime soon. If she could just be reassured that Noah was well, she could better endure their separation.

In her mind, she revisited the scant memories she'd had with her son. Birthing him. Nursing him. Talking to him when her folks were out of hearing. The painful day she'd told him goodbye stood out most prevalent.

He'd been too young to understand heartbreak, and Lily was glad for that. But her own misery was impossible to bear. Her ma had whisked him away from her so fast, Lily hadn't had time to cherish him.

Unable to help herself, she sobbed harder.

Everyone told her over and over again that she was a strong woman. But for today, she intended to allow herself one small weakness.

Noah . . .

* * *

A persistent rap on the door woke Lily from a restless slumber.

Her head pounded. She'd cried for hours and couldn't remember falling asleep. Now she had to pay the price for shedding so many tears.

She sniffled and rubbed her sore eyes. "Yes?"

"Miss Larsen?" Jenny's soft voice held such compassion, it touched Lily to the core. "Can we come in?"

"Just a minute." She scooted into a seated position and pulled the blankets around her. "All right. You can come in now." Surely, she must look a sight, but at the moment, she didn't care.

Jenny walked in followed by . . .

Oh, my.

Lily gasped.

Arabelle was sitting in her wheelchair, being pushed by Winnie. Lily had been unable to convince her to get in the thing ever since her first attempt at putting her there. Yet she rolled in wearing a soft smile, seemingly comfortable.

Levi and Opal trailed in behind Winnie, grinning as if on an adventure.

Lily held a hand to her heart. "How . . .?"

Arabelle's smile grew. "My girls helped me into the chair. You've done so much for me, Lily, and it seems for once I can do something for you. And since you allowed us to enter, I assume you're not contagious. Otherwise, I know you would've cautioned us to keep our distance."

"Of course, I would." Lily clutched her belly and burst into another fit of sobs.

Why am I bein' such a baby?

She covered her face with her hands, embarrassed for making such a scene.

"Winnie?" Arabelle said. "Move me beside the bed, then take Levi and the others to play, so I can speak with Miss Larsen alone. All right?"

"Yes, Mother." Winnie did exactly what had been asked of her. And when all the children were out of the room, she shut the door tight.

"Talk to me, Lily." Arabelle rested a hand on Lily's arm. The movement alone was an enormous step forward. Every day she'd gotten stronger, and she hadn't stopped thanking Lily for pushing her.

They'd been getting along well, and Lily had started seeing her as more of a friend than an employer. But she wasn't sure if she was ready to fully open up and tell her secrets.

"Lily?" Arabelle persisted. "You're not truly ill, are you?"

"I'm sick inside, but it's nothin' a doctor can fix."

"So, tell me. What's troubling you?"

Lily doubled over and rocked back and forth. "I'm afraid you'll think poorly of me if I tell you."

Arabelle gently rubbed Lily's back. "I'd never think badly of the person who brought me back to life. It might make you feel better to talk about what's making you cry. And whatever you say will stay between us. I promise."

Lily rose and pressed her palm against her aching chest.

Arabelle gave her the saddest look, then sat back and gripped the arms of her chair. "Someone broke your heart, didn't they?"

Lily nodded.

"A man, I assume?"

Another nod. It was simpler than speaking.

"Is that why you went to Water's Rest? Did he molest you?"

Lily gaped at her. "Heavens, no. I loved him. But . . ." Her chin vibrated and more tears streamed.

"Go on . . ."

"We planned to marry. It's a long horrible story I won't trouble you with. For now, all you need to know is why I'm cryin'. I let him go an' I've done all I can to wash away his memory. But . . ." She took a deep breath and kept her eyes on Arabelle, worried about how she'd respond. "I had his son. Since we weren't married, I shamed my family. My folks didn't want anyone to know, so they took him from me an' pretended he was theirs. They sent me away to forget him, but I can't."

Lily covered her face and bawled harder than ever. "Today's his birthday." She rasped several large breaths. "He's a year old. I miss him terribly. I wanna see him so bad it makes every bone in my body ache." She lay down and faced the wall, crying.

"Oh, Lily. I'm sorry you've been hurt this way. I can't imagine . . ."

Is she *cryin'?*

Lily slowly twisted around to see her. Arabelle appeared as distraught as Lily felt. "Arabelle? I didn't mean to make *you* cry."

"It's terrible what you've been through. To have your parents treat you that way and make you give up your child. But . . . what happened to the man? The one you loved?"

She searched Lily's face as if her answer would have a direct effect on her. Truthfully, she looked scared to death.

Lily carefully chose her words. "He married someone else."

"Did he know about the child?"

"No. I never told him." There were so many pieces to Lily's puzzled life that had been left out, but she didn't have the strength to tell everything. "It's hard to explain, but I don't blame him for marryin' her. He was a good man, tryin' to do the right thing."

"Right? For him maybe." Arabelle's head dropped low. "Arthur's a good man, too. But even upstanding men can falter." She lifted her chin high and stared blankly as if lost somewhere. Silent tears streamed down her face.

Something truly troubled Arabelle. Had Mr. Jacobson stepped out on her? He certainly didn't seem like the sort of man who'd be unfaithful. No matter, Lily couldn't bring herself to question Arabelle about such a sensitive subject.

Arabelle blinked slowly and faced her. "Men have needs. Since you've had a child, you understand." Once again, her eyes glazed over and she lost all expression. "Every night, I lay motionless in bed beside my husband and wonder what he's thinking. I fear Arthur will look elsewhere for affection and the physical bond I can no longer provide."

Lily sat upright and scooted close to her. "He'd *never* do that. He loves you—thinks the *world* a you. He told me so himself."

"Every woman convinces herself that the man she loves wouldn't put his eyes on anyone but her. Didn't you think *your* man would stay true to *you*?"

"Of course, I did. But our circumstance was quite different."

Arabelle folded her hands atop her lap. "I keep waiting for the day Arthur doesn't come home from work, or arrives smelling of another woman's perfume. He's handsome and successful. I have no doubt there are women with their sights on him. Good men have been scarcer since the war took so many lives."

Lily cupped her hand over Arabelle's. "If you honestly believe there are women hoverin' 'round the general store waitin' to get their wretched claws into your husband, then I'd say you best be gettin' out of the house some. Be seen by his side. You can show the women of Asheville that Arthur Jacobson is taken."

Arabelle turned her head. "By a *cripple*."

Lily's tears had dried. Though tempted to scold Arabelle for wallowing in self-pity, she couldn't. After all, she'd been doing some wallowing, too. At least she could overcome her own worries by focusing on someone else's troubles.

She chose to concentrate on the good in the situation, and not Arabelle's limitations. "*You* hold your husband's heart. You're a beautiful woman who gave him four exceptional children. There are more important things in life than satisfyin' the intimate desires of a man. 'Sides, I think he *is* fulfilled simply by seein' you happy. Your arms have become strong enough to hold him. I'm sure that means everythin' to him."

"But, what if—"

"Stop." Lily held up a hand. "*What ifs* only muddle up happiness. You keep on improvin' the way you have, an' I reckon a day won't go by that your husband won't be wearin' a smile on his face. I believe I've never seen so much love in a man's eyes than what his show for you. He'd do anythin' to make you happy."

Arabelle reached out to Lily. "Thank you." She took hold of Lily's hand and cradled it to her cheek. "I came in to cheer you up and here I am pouring out all *my* woes. Can you forgive me?"

"There's no need to ask it." Lily smiled and brought her hand to herself. "I care 'bout you. Truth be told, I've grown to love your entire family. You've all helped me more than you realize. I was dyin' inside. Someday, I'll hafta tell you 'bout my Aunt Helen. But not today. I'm upset enough as it is."

Arabelle nodded. "Lily?"

"Yes?"

"I know you miss your son, and I'm certain my children can't take his place in your heart. If his father has married someone else, wouldn't *you* like to marry and have a family of your own?"

"I thought so. An' I tried." She blew out a breath. "But that's *another* story."

"My goodness. For someone so young, you've had your share of life." She smiled and tipped her head. "I'll be forever grateful fate brought you here. I hope we'll make a memorable chapter in your life's story."

Lily found herself grinning. Something she hadn't thought possible today. "Only a chapter? Are you sayin' you don't want me to stay forever?"

Arabelle pulled her shoulders back. "Selfishly, I'd love to keep you here. *Always*. But I have a feeling, you'll be on your way to another adventure sooner rather than later."

"Adventure . . ." Lily shut her eyes and pictured Mrs. Gottlieb. "A dear friend a mine used the same word to describe where life would take me. We never really know, do we?"

Arabelle frowned and gestured to the wheelchair. "No, we don't."

Lily threw her covers back, swung her feet onto the floor, then ran her fingers through her mussed hair. "I'm tired a bein' in this room. Why don't you let me wheel you outside today? Get some fresh air?"

"In our nightgowns?" Arabelle's soft laugh put their shared mood back in its proper place.

"Reckon we'd get some strange looks, wouldn't we?"

"Yes. Not to mention, we'd likely freeze."

"Fine. I'll wheel you to your room, help you dress, then I'll put on my fancy blue gown. I know Jenny would love to dress up for a stroll to town, an' she's been dyin' to put one a them pretty hats on your head."

Arabelle worked her lower lip with her teeth. "I want to go, but I'm scared."

"Imagine how surprised your husband will be when he sees us. I think that'll make it worthwhile."

Arabelle didn't argue.

And though Lily's heart still weighed her down, it helped to share part of her secret. Even so, she was grateful that Arabelle didn't ask her Caleb's name, or worse yet, how she currently felt about him. Considering Arabelle felt threatened about some wayward women trying to take her husband away, she wouldn't appreciate knowing that Lily had often thought of attempting to do that very thing to Rebecca.

It was sinful and wrong to even think it. But she'd give almost anything to have him back in her life. For that reason alone, she knew she had to stay away from Waynesville.

Chapter 14

The flames from the fire flickered brightly, but Violet couldn't get warm. She threw on another log, yet no matter how many caught fire, they didn't seem to be producing a lot of heat. Likely because there were too many cracks in the weaner house walls, and icy wind seeped through every tiny space.

She shivered and headed for the bed. At least the covers would help. If her husband would come home, all would be well.

She'd left him in the barn with his pa, where the two were preparing meat for storage. Mrs. Quincy had gathered the neighbors together to butcher hogs. They'd all pitched in and helped, then shared what they'd butchered. Last November at hog-killing time, there were few to be had. But things had greatly improved in the cove.

Violet stayed away from any kind of butchering. She loved to eat meat, but didn't like to think about where it came from. Her ma had always told them that was why butchered pigs were called ham and bacon. That way, they didn't have to say they were eating swine. Just like cows on a plate were steak or burger.

Fish are always fish. Wonder why that is?

She shrugged and burrowed under the covers. Odd how her mind wandered when she was cold. Of course, since she'd stopped fretting about things, she'd often had silly wayward thoughts.

They'd celebrate Thanksgiving in a few days, and she was definitely thankful. Not only for her new family, but most recently, for the long-awaited letter she'd received from Lily.

It eased Violet knowing her sister was well and living with a loving family. But she also felt Lily's pain when she wrote about how much she missed Noah.

Violet had written to her in return, but had taken Gideon's advice and not mentioned how often their ma took Noah to stay at the Henderson's. She didn't want Lily enduring additional hurt from knowing such a thing.

It was comforting to have Lily closer than she'd been when she'd lived in St. Louis. Asheville could be reached in a four-day ride, rather than the weeks it took to get to Missouri. Even so, Violet had no idea how she'd ever be able to get away to see her. She couldn't travel alone, and Gideon had too much to do around the farm, so he couldn't go with her. Besides, winter would soon arrive, and no one would be going *anywhere* till spring.

She sighed. As much as she loved Gideon, and as good a friend as he'd become, no one could replace Lily.

"Thank goodness for letters," she mumbled and pulled the blankets up over her head.

* * *

"Thank you!" Lily hugged the precious letter to her breast. She instantly recognized Violet's handwriting.

Mr. Jacobson chuckled. "Why don't you take some time and go to the privacy of your room to read it. Supper can wait."

Lily nearly burst into happy tears. "Thank you." She curtsied, then hurried to her bedroom and shut the door. The sound of the children's laughter followed her.

Yes, she'd acted a bit unusual, but she'd gladly take their teasing. She'd been anxiously awaiting the arrival of some sort of news from the cove, and most importantly, word about Noah.

She carefully unsealed the envelope, even though she'd been tempted to rip it open.

Unable to be still, she paced and read.

Dear Lily,

I cried when I got your letter. I had been worrying myself sick wondering where you might be. All Aunt Helen told us in the hateful letter she sent was that she had put you out in the streets where you belonged. It was a horrid thing for her to say, but nothing coming from her truly surprises me. She's a wretched woman.

I know we are supposed to love our relatives, but I despise her for the way she treated you. Relative or not.

Lily flopped down onto her bed. She didn't like to think about the months with Aunt Helen, but she hated that she'd caused Violet so much worry.

She should've at least sent a telegram from Water's Rest to let Violet know she was well. But at the time, she wasn't. If she'd been herself and her mind had been right, she would've had the sense to contact her sister. Hopefully one day, she'd be able to ask for Violet's forgiveness, face-to-face.

Lily lay on her back and lifted the letter.

I thank God every day for Gideon. If not for my husband, I think I would go mad. He reassured me that you were fine and reminded me of your strength and resolve. It helped to hear it, but you know me. I always think the worst thoughts.

Now that I know you're safe and with a loving family, I can rest easier. It's wonderful that you are tending four children. You spoke of each of them with such fondness. I can tell they have worked their way into your heart.

It must be hard to look at little Levi and not think of Noah. This past year has flown by so quickly, and it makes me sad that you have missed the many things he has already done. I wish you could come home and take him away with you. It's probably wrong of me to say it, but I believe that children should be with whoever loves them the most. He should be with you.

Lily shut her eyes and breathed deeply. She and Violet had always been truthful with each other, but honesty like this hurt. And since they knew each other so well, Lily was certain it had been hard for Violet to write the words.

What had compelled her to do it? Were their folks treating him poorly?

Lily didn't want to consider such a thing. Perhaps if she finished the letter, she'd get a better understanding.

Noah is walking everywhere, and has been for a while now. His legs are still chubby, but eventually, I imagine he will be as skinny as Horace.

Ma gave Noah his first haircut some time ago. He is more adorable than ever. I swear he is the prettiest baby boy I have ever seen. It shouldn't surprise me. Not when he has such a lovely ma.

"An' *pa*," Lily mumbled.

I haven't mentioned this to anyone yet—not even Gideon—but I may be with child. I expected my flow the end of October and here it is November the twelfth and it still has not arrived. If nothing happens by Christmas, I will give the news to Gideon as a gift. Just the thought of having his child has brought me happiness.

Lily's heart leapt for her sister, but a hint of jealousy crept in. Violet was living the kind of life that Lily desired. Worse yet, Lily would give anything to be there to share this with her. She'd always believed they'd rear their children close enough to each other that the cousins could play and holiday celebrations would be huge and joyful.

As she'd told Arabelle, no one ever knew where their life would take them. But Lily had always thought she'd have some say in the matter.

Gideon and I would like to have a large family. We hope that our children will help heal his folks. They don't talk about it much, but I know they miss their other boys. Gideon misses them, too. Our family was luckier than most families in the war. Pa could have easily been killed, and if the war had lasted longer, surely Lucas would have had to fight. Although, we both know he wanted to.

As for Lucas, Pa showed me a telegram that Mr. Douglas sent from Knoxville. They are staying with Mrs. Ableman. The message was short and simple, as are all telegrams. All we know is that they are trying to decide where to go from there in search of Callie.

If the poor widow knew of Lucas's deceit, she would probably have him jailed for fraud. He would deserve it for using money that wasn't rightfully his.

I often wonder if we will ever see Lucas again. Sadly, I don't miss him one bit. You, however, I long for every day. Thank goodness we can write to each other now. Please keep me abreast of everything you do. It's wonderful that you're helping the Jacobsons. I cannot imagine what it must be like for Mrs. Jacobson to lose the use of both her legs.

I witnessed how distraught Gideon was over losing one leg. He was so full of anger when I saw him the first time that I feared I would never get through to him. I thought of you and asked myself what you would do in my situation, and I approached him fearlessly. There is a lot of self-gratification that comes from helping someone else become the best they can be. But more than that, it lifts my heart seeing him happy.

I imagine you feel that way about Arabelle. (Such a lovely name.) As much as I wish you were here with me, I understand that you are where you need to be. They are blessed to have you.

It is impossible to say what our futures hold, but I know one thing for sure. I want you to share mine, even if it has to be in correspondence alone.

I am so lucky to be able to call you my sister.

I love you forever,

Violet

Tears filled Lily's eyes and spilled onto her cheeks.

"I love you, too."

She stood and wandered to the window. In another month, the ground would be covered in snow.

Somehow, come spring, she'd find a way to go home. Even if it was only for a visit, she had to see Violet, and of course, her sweet baby boy.

* * *

Caleb set aside the pitchfork, folded his arms, and simply listened. When his ma got this particular tone in her voice, he couldn't do much more.

"I'm serious 'bout this, Caleb." His ma's eyes pinched into slits. "You should be watchin' her closer. Sumthin' ain't right."

He took a breath and prayed he'd say the right words. "She's fine, Ma. Happy as can be. Ever since I built that swing, she's been on it every afternoon. Less it rains. Mostly, she gets on it when Avery's nappin'."

"Swingin' don't do nothin' for her health. If anythin', she'll catch cold out there in the wind. What were you thinkin' puttin' that thing up with winter nearly upon us?"

Caleb huffed and shook his head. Seemed he'd never please his ma in regard to Rebecca. Even when he'd done something that made his wife happy. "She *likes* the swing. You shoulda seen her face the first time I showed it to her. She was like the Becca I knew when we was kids. Carefree an' gay. Beautiful, too."

His ma stepped closer and pointed a finger in his face. "She's gettin' too thin. Understand me? Any thinner an' she'll blow away while she's swingin'. Ain't she got nothin' better to do with her time than play 'round like a child?"

"No." He braced a hand against the wall of the barn. "You know full well I do all the work 'round here. Course, she does the household chores an' watches Avery, but that don't take a lotta time."

"No needlework?"

"Uh-uh. She made them curtains for the house when we first moved in, but hasn't sewed a stitch since. This here shirt has a button what come off. I just go without it."

"What 'bout your socks? Does she darn?"

"Nope. If I took my boot off, you'd see. My big toe will likely freeze an' fall off come winter."

His ma smacked his shoulder. "Don't talk like that."

"Every sock I own needs mendin'. But I don't wanna pester her 'bout fixin' 'em. I love her, Ma. She's a good woman . . ."

"But . . .?" Again, her eyes narrowed. "C'mon, I can hear that *but* in there."

"But she ain't cut out to be the wife of a farmer. The other day, she told me again how she wishes we could live at the hotel. Then, she went out an' got on that swing."

His ma looked directly at him. "You ain't still pinin' over that Larsen woman, are you? Thinkin' *she'd* be the perfect farmer's wife?"

"No." She cautiously eyed him, so he persisted. "I *swear* it, Ma. I ain't thought 'bout Lily in a long while. Becca an' me's doin' fine. Regardless of my holey socks. You worry too much."

"Only cuz I love you both." She stepped back, shaking her head. "I still say she's too thin. Did you tell her I invited you to Thanksgivin' dinner at the hotel?"

"Yep. An' she's thrilled. She was afraid she'd burn the turkey. She's gonna bake a couple pumpkin pies."

"Good. An' I'll make sure she eats several pieces. With cream, too. Anythin' I can do to fatten her up." His ma walked toward the barn door. "Don't stay out here too long. You need to spend some a your day with your family."

"I'm 'bout done. Just cleanin' things up."

"Well, I best be goin'. Gotta get back to the hotel 'fore it gets dark."

Caleb strode across the barn floor and hugged her. "Thanks for comin' by. We appreciate the bacon you brought. I'm glad Becca knows how to cook it. I can look forward to a fine breakfast in the mornin'."

"You're welcome. I'll see you Thursday. They'll be servin' the meal at three o'clock."

"We'll be there."

She kissed his cheek, then crinkled her nose and wiped her mouth. "Goodness, you've been sweatin'. Ain't you?"

"Yep. Didn't ask you to kiss me." He grinned. "Don't worry, Ma. I'll take a bath 'fore I kiss on my girls."

She stood tall. "Least I raised you right." Finally, she smiled. The warm, loving kind of smile he'd carried with him into battle. "I love you, son."

"I love you, too, Ma."

Her smile softened, then she walked away.

Caleb leaned against the wall.

Thanksgivin'.

Fond memories of hunting the buck with Lily and Lucas came to mind. They'd eaten well that Thanksgiving. No, he hadn't thought of Lily in a while, but it seemed she managed to creep into his memories every now and then.

And Lucas . . .

If the boy wasn't dead by now, he was certainly up to no good.

Maybe I did *do wrong by him.*

If he'd paid more attention to the boy, perhaps he wouldn't have gone astray. But whether Caleb did wrong or right, he couldn't change the past.

He had to be thankful for the present and hope for a better future.

Chapter 15

Lily stood back and smiled. "My goodness. You're as lovely as a picture."

Arabelle looked downward. "Tell me the truth. Am I fine enough to go into town? Will people gawk at me?"

"If they do, it'll be because you're beautiful."

The children gathered at Lily's side, beaming with pride. Except for Levi. Lily had to keep grabbing onto him to stop him from climbing into his ma's lap.

"The hat I chose is perfect," Jenny said. "The red ribbon matches the trim of your dress."

Winnie gave her sister a slightly jealous-looking sideways glance, then returned her attention to her ma. "She's right, Mother. And even though you'll be wearing your winter coat, the red will show beneath it."

Opal giggled. "Father will be surprised."

"Papa?" Levi's face screwed together.

Lily took the opportunity to lift Levi from the floor and hold him close. "We're gonna go see him at work. But we all gotta bundle up real good."

"That's right," Arabelle said. "I don't want any of you catching cold. You'll need to wear your scarves and gloves along with your coats. If we're fortunate, we'll see some Christmas decorations.

Your father mentioned that some of the businesses were decorating the town center, as well as their own buildings."

"Christmas!" Opal clapped her hands. "Soon, we'll hang our stockings for Santa Claus." She tugged on Lily's sleeve. "Do you know about Santa?"

"Saint Nicholas," Lily said, smiling. "I've heard stories. But I reckon he never knew 'bout our cabin in the cove. Even so, I know all 'bout Christmas. My ma read us the nativity story every year an' we celebrated Jesus' birthday. When we were able, we exchanged presents. But no matter, it was a happy time. 'Specially at church."

Winnie knelt beside her ma. "Can *we* go to church this year? I love the Christmas music."

Arabelle reached out and stroked Winnie's cheek. "We'll see how I'm feeling. All right?"

"Yes, Mother." Winnie stood tall and nodded at the coatrack. "Let's go so we have plenty of time to visit Father. I'd like to look around the store to see what I want for Christmas."

Jenny jutted her chin high. "I already got *my* gift."

"You did?"

"Yes." She placed a hand on her ma's shoulder. "I got to dress Mother in a fancy hat."

Arabelle smiled and patted Jenny's hand. "Yes, you did. But I'm sure there's something else you'd like to find for yourself under the tree Christmas morning."

Jenny sighed and her shoulders slumped. "There *is* something, but I don't know if it would be right to ask for it."

"It can't hurt to ask. That's what's special about Christmas."

Jenny gazed upward as if trying to decide what to say, but her lips remained sealed. Lily couldn't imagine what the girl might want. Perhaps when the time was right, Lily would ask her.

Levi squirmed in Lily's arms and reached for his ma.

Arabelle's soft laughter was as lovely as Arabelle herself. "I can take him, Lily. He can ride on my lap into town."

Though it pleased Lily to see the bond that had developed between the two, a small part of her hated to give him up. Regardless, she placed him on his ma's lap.

It had to be odd not being able to feel him against her legs, but then again, the instant the boy put his arms around Arabelle, Lily knew she could feel his hugs. The glow on her face said more than words.

"All right." Lily gestured to the door. "Bundle up an' let's go. I'll push your ma. Winnie an' Jenny, you each hold one a Opal's hands."

They obeyed without question.

It was quite a long stroll to the general store, but the cold air had frozen the ground, so Lily easily pushed the wheelchair. The children's excitement surely kept them plenty warm. More so than their clothes.

As for Arabelle, it had taken a while to get her to agree to go out. Even after she'd expressed concern over the possibility of other women taking a shine to her husband. But Lily hadn't given up. She hadn't nagged Arabelle, but ever-so-often, she'd gently suggest an outing. Perhaps the Christmas spirit had taken hold of her and made her agreeable today.

Every day since Lily's arrival, Arabelle had grown more comfortable in her own skin. Lily could tell by the way she reacted to simply being bathed and groomed. Her poor attitude had vanished, and she'd become strong enough to clean herself and even wash her own body in the bathtub. Of course, it took both Lily and Winnie to get her *into* the tub, and Lily was always close by, in case her dear friend lost her balance.

In a little over a month's time, Arabelle felt more like a sister to Lily, rather than someone she worked for.

The three girls skipped along the road and sang a song unfamiliar to Lily. It had silly repetitive words, but they sang with such joy that they drew looks from many passersby.

Arabelle craned her neck and looked back at Lily. "I owe their happiness to you."

"Me?" Lily kept pushing. "You should give yourself credit. They came to life when you did."

"But I never would have, if you'd not come into our home. I owe you a great deal."

Lily stopped, readjusted her scarf to fully cover her neck, then started pushing again. "Your husband pays me plenty. 'Sides, you made me part a your family. That's priceless."

Winnie whipped around and faced them, wide-eyed. "Do you see all the boughs and red ribbons?"

"Yes, I do." Arabelle said.

The three girls squealed with excitement and hurried even faster down the road.

"Don't run!" Lily called out after them, but they kept going.

"They're fine," Arabelle said. "We're nearly there. Winnie will take them to the store and we can scold them when we catch up to them." She laughed. "Of course, by the time we arrive, Arthur will likely have given them all sweets, and they'll be impossible."

Levi's head popped up. "Sweets?"

"I promise, you'll get some, too."

He burrowed against her and shut his eyes.

"Lily?" Arabelle once again glanced upward. Her voice no longer held laughter.

"Yes?"

"I'm trying my best not to worry about Arthur becoming dissatisfied with me. I hope I'm making a step in the right direction —so to speak." She lowered her head and tightened her grasp around Levi.

"You are. When he sees you, he's gonna light up like a Christmas tree."

"I hope so. Of course, with the girls going on ahead, it won't be much of a surprise."

"No matter." Lily stopped and knelt beside her. "I reckon he hasn't seen you dressed up so fine since before the accident. Am I right?"

Arabelle nodded.

"Then it *will* be a surprise. You ain't in your nightgown."

Arabelle's head tipped to one side. "Every now and then, your English slips. I have a feeling you have more stories to tell me, Lily Larsen."

"That I do. But not today. I'll try harder to speak proper." She grinned, stood erect, and pushed the wheelchair up the ramp at the side of the store. A blessed convenience put there to help vendors wheel in their goods.

Unlike the first time Lily entered the store, it was abuzz with numerous customers. She spied Mrs. Wood, who continued to flourish from the laundry the Jacobsons created every week. The woman had a basket on her arm that she was filling with all sorts of items—from canned goods to Christmas candles.

"Do you see Arthur?" Arabelle craned her neck. "I feel like I've become a small child again unable to see around all the goods."

"Well . . ." Lily held a hand to her heart. "*He's* seen *you*." She turned the wheelchair so Arabelle could face her husband.

Mr. Jacobson had withdrawn a handkerchief from his pocket and was dabbing at his eyes. "Arabelle?" He nearly stumbled over a customer, blinded by tears.

"Hello, Arthur." Her chin trembled. She, too, was about to cry.

The overwhelming emotion had an effect on Lily as well. Her throat dried and she had to put her back to the scene to keep her own tears from falling. She wanted this kind of love.

"Papa!" Levi's sweet voice turned Lily's head. He squirmed from Arabelle's lap and soon was in his pa's arms.

Even while holding the child, the man hadn't taken his eyes off Arabelle. "You're so beautiful." He lightly touched her hat. "I remember when I bought this for you."

"Jenny selected it over all my others and insisted I wear it. She helped with my hair, too."

He went down on one knee, with Levi still clinging to him. "I saw the girls come in and expected Miss Larsen, but . . ." Again, he wiped his eyes. "Oh, Arabelle. I'm so proud of you."

She put a hand to his cheek and he cradled it there. Lily would never forget this moment.

"Mrs. Jacobson?" A loud gray-haired woman disrupted the tender couple. She pushed past several others to reach them. "Arabelle, is that you?"

"Hello, Mrs. Tierney."

"My goodness, dear. You're looking quite well. And . . ." She gingerly touched the wheelchair. "You're out of bed."

Arabelle sat tall in the chair. "Yes, I am. As are you." She smiled broadly.

"Well, of course *I* am." The woman let out an obnoxious laugh. "You meant that to be humorous, didn't you?"

"Yes. I did."

The woman pursed her wrinkled lips. "You're most definitely not the same woman I cared for all those months ago. But I'm happy to see it. Will you be attending worship?"

Mr. Jacobson guided the old woman away from his wife. "Perhaps. We'll see how Arabelle is feeling. Now, is there anything in particular you wish to purchase today?"

"Actually, there is."

"Good." He led her even farther away. Fortunately, Levi didn't complain and held on tight.

"My," Lily mumbled. "She was sumthin'. She must be one a them church women who tended you."

"Yes. She's a dear, but can be a bit much. Thank goodness for Arthur."

"As I told you, your husband is a wonderful man. Did you see those tears in his eyes when he saw you? If that's not love, I don't know what is."

Arabelle reached for Lily's hand. "Forgive me for implying anything bad about him. Please? He hasn't done one thing to make me question his behavior. Fear plays horrid games on the mind."

Lily grasped her hand and squeezed. "Yes, it does. An' I've decided to stop bein' afraid myself. Come spring, I'm goin' home no matter what the outcome. I hafta find out sumthin' 'bout my son an' how my folks are treatin' him. I'm his ma, an' it's up to me to make sure he's raised proper."

"What if you find he's not?"

"Then I reckon there'll be a new resident in Asheville."

"You'd bring him back with you?"

Lily shut her eyes and pictured the last time she'd held him. "In a heartbeat."

She smiled and warmth spread all the way to her cold toes. Spring would arrive soon enough and she'd face whatever came her way.

Chapter 16

The fresh pine boughs Lily had placed on the mantel gave the entire house a refreshing clean smell. Soon, Mr. Jacobson and the children would be coming in with a Christmas tree that would add even more outdoor scent. The children would surely be cold, but they'd all asked to go with him to select just the right tree.

Later in the evening, they planned to pop some corn to make garland. Only the older girls would be allowed to use needles to thread it, but Lily knew everyone would enjoy eating it.

Arabelle sat in her wheelchair in the corner of the living room, trying to tat some lace for the girls' Christmas dresses. She huffed and dropped her hands onto her lap. "It's no use. It's too hard."

The intricate work was her biggest challenge yet.

Lily had noticed frustration working its way onto Arabelle's face. But she didn't want to discourage her from trying. She'd never do that. "Why don't you set it aside for a spell? I can fix you a cup a cider."

"This used to be so easy." Arabelle let the ivory shuttle fall to the floor, along with a large amount of thread.

Whether or not it had been intentional didn't matter to Lily. She picked up the items and examined them closely. "I doubt I could do this myself. Even with two strong hands. It looks complicated."

Arabelle cast a half-smile. "As I said, it used to be easy for me. Would you like me to show you how it works?" She gestured to the shuttle.

Lily sat at the end of the sofa, close to her wheelchair. "You can show me, but I doubt I'll be able to do it."

"Now who's being negative?" Arabelle grinned.

Lily smirked and rolled her eyes, then held up the items. "Fine. Tell me what to do?"

"You wrap the thread around your left hand, and you work the shuttle with your right. The hook on the end is what catches the thread and makes the loops that form the lace."

"Mercy, it sounds difficult."

"Here. I'll show you." Arabelle reached for the items and demonstrated exactly what she'd explained, making it look easy.

"Arabelle." Lily watched every move she made. "You're doin' it."

Within moments, Arabelle had formed a perfect loop. She stared at it, then shook her head. "I don't understand. I kept trying and . . ." She laughed. "It worked." With renewed energy, she started again. Her hands flew as if they had their own mind, remembering exactly what they had to do.

Lily sat back and admired the piece as it formed into a more intricate design. She wouldn't dream of stopping her now for more lessons. The dear woman was making incredible progress.

The door opened and with it came a gust of cold air and excited chatter.

"Trismas tree!" Levi shouted and ran across the room to them.

Lily grabbed hold of him before he got tangled in his ma's thread. "Did your pa chop one down?"

The boy pointed at the open door.

"Is it as tall as you?" Lily tickled his belly.

Levi giggled. "Big tree." He threw his arms up high above his head.

Mr. Jacobson hauled in the large pine. He'd already placed a cross-cut wood stand in front of the living room window. Winnie and Jenny helped him wiggle the tree into place. Opal stood back, grinning. Her cold, bright-red nose didn't seem to be bothering her.

Lily couldn't recall the last time her family had a Christmas tree. Her ma always said it was wasteful and senseless to kill a tree, simply to decorate and fawn over it. She'd said that if anyone wanted to appreciate a pine, all they had to do was take a walk through the woods.

Mr. Jacobson stepped out from behind the tree, sniffing his hands. He repetitively touched his index finger to his thumb. They looked as though they were sticking together. "A little pitchy. I best go wash." He stopped in the middle of the floor and gaped at Arabelle, whose hands hadn't quit moving. "You're *tatting*."

Smiling, she lifted her eyes. "Yes, I am." Without skipping a beat, she kept on going.

He beamed. "Girls, your mother is *tatting*."

Opal giggled. "You already said that, Father."

His grin didn't fade. He wandered off to the kitchen, happily mumbling. The two older girls followed him, chattering that they also needed to wash.

Arabelle giggled in a manner that sounded a lot like Opal. "I believe he doubted I could do this," she whispered to Lily.

Only minutes prior, someone else had doubted it, too, but Lily wouldn't point that out. The mood in the house was too joyful to douse.

Mr. Jacobson returned, wiping his hands on a towel. He patted his coat pocket. "I have something for you, Lily."

"For me?"

He pulled out two envelopes and handed them to her. "It would seem there are a number of people who miss you."

Her heart pattered harder. It hadn't been long since she'd gotten Violet's letter. She doubted she'd get another one from her so soon. She gnawed her lower lip and looked closely at each one.

The first, she recognized, and it tugged at her insides.

Pa.

The other, she wasn't certain of, but it was postmarked in St. Louis. That meant it could be a number of people. However, the penmanship wasn't Mrs. Gottlieb's.

"Don't you want to read them?" Arabelle asked.

"Course I do." She gulped. "Reckon I'll go to my room."

Lily stood and Mr. Jacobson took her place on the sofa beside his wife.

They said nothing as she walked away, went into her bedroom, and shut the door.

Good news or bad news?

The inanimate pieces of paper in her hand churned her belly.

Perhaps it was silly to become anxious over correspondence, but she recalled how a single letter had changed her life forever.

Assuming the letter from St. Louis must be from someone she cared for, she set her pa's aside. She feared what he might say.

Maybe Archibald—her dear caterpillar—had written. If so, why hadn't he put a return address on the face of the envelope?

She carefully opened the letter and spread the pages smooth.

22 November, 1866

Dear Lily,

Once you realize who this letter is from, I fear you won't finish reading, but I pray that you will.

Her mind spun. The unfamiliar handwriting had her perplexed. She quickly flipped to the last page and gasped.

Zachary Danforth

Her stomach churned harder. She'd truly cared for him, but he'd shamed her. He'd spoken so hatefully after she'd poured her heart out to him, then walked away from her and repeated all she'd told him to her uncle. Things she'd prayed would stay private between Zachary and her were spread faster than Mrs. Quincy's gossip.

Her fist slowly tightened around the letter. Why would she care to read anything he had to say?

She flopped down on her bed and stared blankly at the walls. Conflicted, she'd not yet fully crumpled the paper that lay in her hand.

Zachary couldn't possibly want her back in his life. Could he?

She sat up. "No," she whispered. "His folks would never allow it."

Perhaps he intended to shame her further. Maybe he'd put all his hateful feelings in writing.

With a loud huff, she once again smoothed the paper. She wasn't about to be intimidated by a simple letter.

"All right, Zachary," she mumbled. "Tell me what's on your mind."

She wiggled around on the bed till she got comfortable, then breathed deeply and lifted the letter in front of her face.

I don't expect you to forgive me for my behavior on the night we parted.

"You got that right."

However, I will ask it of you nonetheless. Please, forgive me, Lily. I was foolish.

Nothing like what she'd expected to read. It helped knowing she wasn't about to be demeaned again, and her heart eased somewhat.

She continued.

I have always been proud of my intellect. Book learning and sophisticated study comes easy to me. And since I'm being truthful, I confess I can be somewhat of a braggart. I boast of my exceptional academics and pursuit of a medical degree. I rave about my outstanding test scores and relish my father's praise.

All that being said, I acted a fool in regard to you. You opened your heart to me and I pierced it with hateful words.

I was smitten with you. Not only your beauty enthralled me, but your quick wit and intellect as well. You enraptured me in a way no woman ever had. I wanted you in my life. I envisioned our future in a fine home with half a dozen children at our feet, and felt confident that you would be an exceptional mother. I believed that nothing could harm my plans for our lives.

Perhaps that is why I reacted as I did. You managed to mar what I believed was an unblemished plan. That wretched night, I stopped viewing the woman I had fallen in love with and only beheld the acts you had committed. In my mind, your actions ruined everything.

Yes, you had loved before and that foolish man broke your heart.

I should have comforted you, and yet I brought on even more heartache.

And yes, you bore the man's child. A son who was taken from you.

I should have used every possible means I had to help you get him back.

Instead, I destroyed everything. I lost the one woman I know could have made me happy.

It might make you smile to know that Archibald Jones has beaten me up on several occasions. Not physically, of course. He's much too fine a man to behave in that manner. But his words have torn me to shreds. He saw what I had seen in you. Sweet, sweet Lily. A beautiful flower. A precious gem.

I was grateful when Mrs. Gottlieb told me how to reach you. She, too, gave me a piece of her mind. If you haven't heard from her as of yet, you soon will. She misses you a great deal.

Lily stopped reading. Tears had worked their way into her eyes.

She dug into her nightstand drawer and withdrew a hankie. After wiping her eyes and soundly blowing her nose, she returned to the letter.

Mrs. Gottlieb made me swear that I wouldn't say anything hateful to you. I promised her that my letter would be an apology and by no means would I write something cruel. She told me that an honorable man would never have had to pen such a letter. I know very well what she meant. Fortunately, she went on to say that we all make mistakes, and the most important thing we can do is learn from them. She is a very wise woman.

I pray you are well and that you have found a home where you are loved as you should be. I know it's too late for us, and as Archibald reminded me, it would be unfair to even consider asking you to come back to a place where you've been shunned and shamed. I care too much about you to allow that. But my home is here, and honestly, I'm not good enough for you. You deserve someone who sees you for who you are and never questions your goodness or intentions.

I hope you find that someone.

As for me, I doubt I will ever find another Lily.

For now, I will focus solely on my studies and do what I can to become the best doctor possible. A far humbler physician than the one I would have been had I not met you.

Be well. Perhaps someday our lives will bring us together again. If not, I will always think fondly of you and pray you find the utmost happiness.

With love and sincerity,
Zachary Danforth

Lily rubbed her throat to soothe it. Zachary's words should be comforting, but they pained her. Her heart tightened, sending emotions every which way. He truly loved her. If only he'd realized it sooner.

They could've had a future together that would've included Noah. Zachary had said so.

She pinched her eyes firmly shut.

Why? I don't understand why nothin' ever goes right for me. Why, God?

It made no sense to keep being led down dead-end roads.

"Lily?" Mr. Jacobson rapped at her door. "Are you all right?"

She sniffled. "I'm fine."

"Are you certain?"

"Yes." She didn't like to lie, but she also didn't care to talk about it. Lying was easier. "I'll be out in a little while."

"Very well. Let us know if you need anything."

"Thank you. I will."

She fell onto her back and grabbed her pa's letter. If she was going to have an all-out bawl, she might as well put more fuel on her fire.

He had horrible handwriting, but she'd always been able to make out what her ma referred to as *chicken scratches.*

Dear Lily,

It's been a dog's age since I seen you.

The crops is good. Ain't rained as much as we need, but we're getting by.

Your ma don't know I'm writing this. But after talking to your sister, I knew I should say something to you.

I'm sure by now you know all about Mrs. Henderson keeping Noah.

Lily reread the last line, then shook her head in disbelief. Violet hadn't said a word about Mrs. Henderson. Why on earth would *she* be keeping him?

As I explained to Violet, your ma ain't doing too good. Her mind ain't right. She's forgetful and hateful most of the time. If you saw her today, I doubt you'd recognize her.

Violet told me I should take her to a doctor. Reckon I will come spring. I keep hoping she'll wake up one morning like her old self. The Rose I knew before the war.

I started leaving Noah with Mrs. Henderson shortly after Violet and Gideon got married. Violet had been looking after the boy when she lived here with us. Now that she's a wife, she has other responsibilities. Sides, your ma and me don't want Noah thinking Violet's his ma. We don't want him confused.

Every breath Lily took came faster and faster. Her head felt light and she struggled to stay upright.

"My poor baby . . ." She blubbered out unstoppable tears, then tried to wipe them away so she could finish reading.

She had nothing bad to say about Mrs. Henderson. She'd always been a decent woman, but Noah was so little that he might start thinking *she* was his ma.

Spring couldn't come soon enough.

She rubbed her eyes and breathed slowly through her nose, then returned to the letter.

Don't worry none about your boy. He's growing big and strong. I make sure he has plenty to eat and clean clothes to wear.

I'm sorry things is the way they is. You might think we don't care none about you, but I love you. You're my girl and always will be.

Truth be told, this farm ain't been as productive with you gone. The way you work puts my farm hands to shame. I ain't never seen anyone work so hard. Woman or not. Even when you was a little girl you coulda bested any a them men.

The cove ain't the same anymore. Our home is empty without you in it.

I wish I could ask you to come back, but I can't. Folks wouldn't understand. Sides that, it would be too hard on Noah. I know you. You'd want to step in as his ma, and you know that can't happen. We put things into play that can't be changed. We made our choices and we hafta live with them.

I hope them folks in Asheville is treating you good. They better realize what a fine girl they got.

Love,

Pa

Lily lay face down on her bed and tried to stifle the sound of her sobbing. She'd been torn into pieces all over again. Her pa said their house was empty without her, but didn't want her back again. All to save the family name.

"Lily?" Mr. Jacobson knocked at her door. He sounded more persistent than before.

How could she face him, or Arabelle, or even the children like this? They were having a good time enjoying their Christmas preparations. She'd ruin it for them if she didn't compose herself.

She wiped her entire wet face with one of her blankets. "Yessir?"

"We can hear you crying. Did you receive bad news?"

She bawled harder.

Ever-so-slowly, the door inched open.

Arabelle rolled herself in, then pushed the door shut again. A sight that both amazed and warmed Lily. Something she needed at the moment.

She sat up, but covered her face with her hands and kept on sobbing.

Arabelle moved closer. "Would you like to tell me about it?"

Lily nodded into her hands, then gradually lowered them. "While I . . . try . . . to stop cryin', read these." She extended the tear-stained letters to her friend.

Arabelle silently read. When she finished both, she lay them on the bed and waited without saying a word.

It took Lily some time, but eventually, she blurted out all her feelings and told Arabelle every detail about Zachary, and Archibald, and horrid Aunt Helen. Once Lily finished pouring through the details, her heart had lifted.

"No matter what your father told you," Arabelle said. "Don't change your mind about going to the cove in the spring. Understand?"

Lily grasped onto Arabelle's hand. "You don't hafta worry 'bout that. My mind was made up before I got Pa's letter, an' *nothin'* will change it."

"Good girl." She peered into Lily's eyes. "I know I should've asked your permission to speak of him, but I told Arthur about your son."

Lily cast a reassuring smile. "I assumed you would. Married folks as close as you two seem to talk 'bout everythin'. Just how it should be. Honestly, I'm glad. I always worried that he thought I was a prostitute. I know his sister was, an' it probably wouldn't have bothered him if *I* was, but it troubled me thinkin' he thought that." She fluttered her hands in the air. "I'm ramblin' now, aren't I?"

"A bit." Arabelle grinned. "But what I wanted you to know is that Arthur and I discussed the arrangements in detail. If you'd like to bring Noah here, he's more than welcome. I'm sure Levi would appreciate the playmate."

Lily flung her arms around Arabelle. "Thank you."

If the mountains weren't so dangerous this time of year, Lily would leave immediately.

However, her sensibility would keep her in Asheville a few more months.

Chapter 17

Gideon squeezed Violet's hand. Their heads were bowed in prayer, but his eyes were open. And when she glanced sideways at him and smiled, he felt like the luckiest man in Tennessee. Maybe even the entire country.

"Amen," Brother Davis said, and the congregation repeated, "Amen."

The preacher clutched his Bible to his chest and smiled. "I wish each an' every one of you a blessed Christmas. Let's all join in singin' Silent Night."

Gideon moved his lips, but didn't squeak out even a peep. He wanted to listen to Violet's beautiful voice as she sang with heartfelt passion.

His ma had helped him with Violet's gift. A lavender-colored dress, fitting of her name, complete with a matching hat. Her cheeks had a glow to them he'd not seen before. Christmas had a way of bringing out the best in folks. And since his lovely wife was already the finest woman he knew, the joy of the season made her shine like an angel.

She'd sewn him a sharp white shirt, and gave him store-bought black braces to keep his pants up. She'd mentioned another gift he'd receive later when they were alone.

He chuckled at the thought, having a darn good idea that she'd gift him with some sort of affection. Honestly, Violet never had to give him another thing. Her love was all he needed.

"What are you laughin' for?" Violet whispered in his ear. "Don't you like my singin'?"

"Sorry, sweetheart. You know I love your singin', but my mind was elsewhere."

"Shame on you." She pursed her lips and lightly patted his hand. "We're in church, you're supposed to have your thoughts on God, not silly things that cause you to be humored."

He started to reply, but she held a single finger to her lips and hushed him. She faced forward and started singing again.

She might not have scolded him, if she'd known his mind had been on her.

He looked behind him to the back pew, making certain her folks hadn't left in the middle of the service. Her ma had been so unpredictable, it wouldn't have surprised him.

The woman caught his eye and pushed an awkward smile on her lips, then bounced Noah up and down a few times in her arms. At least she'd brought him to church. Surely Violet would want to see him as soon as the service ended.

It was possible that the child was part of the reason for Violet's excessive happiness. Regardless, Gideon loved seeing her like this. He'd do all he could to keep her happy forever.

After singing all the verses of the song, Brother Davis raised his hands heavenward. "Let's all sing the first verse again."

Violet's eyes closed. She lifted her chin high and the words came easily from her lips. Her voice overpowered nearly everyone in the small church.

Brother Davis smiled at her, but she didn't see it. Gideon gave her hand another squeeze. His silent way of telling her he loved her and how much she was appreciated.

Merry Christmas wishes surrounded them once the song ended and the preacher excused them. Folks bustled from the church—most anxious to get home to their family gatherings. Gideon's ma had put a ham in the oven that morning, not to mention she and Violet had spent Christmas Eve baking up a storm. They'd have a wonderful supper.

"Hurry now, Violet." His ma gave her a nudge. "Go on an' see Noah 'fore your folks leave."

"Yes'm." Violet scooted past Gideon faster than he thought possible. She lifted her skirt and raced down the aisle.

Even his folks knew how much the boy meant to her. Though Violet hadn't told them about Noah's real parentage, his folks had seen how involved Violet had been with his upbringing since the day he was born. Gideon and Violet had chosen not to involve them in the intimate details of the situation. Some things seemed better left private.

Gideon followed her down the aisle.

"Ma!" Violet hollered out. "Pa!"

Her ma kept walking, but her pa stopped and faced them.

"Violet." The man dipped his head. "Gideon." Another dip. "Merry Christmas."

"Can't you stop her?" Violet pointed at her ma. "Least let me give Noah a Christmas kiss."

Mr. Larsen's brows drew in, then he turned his head. "Rose! Come over here with our boys!"

The instant he yelled, Horace and Isaac spun on their heels and raced to Violet. Hugs were given all around. Of course, Gideon shook their hands like a proper brother-in-law should.

Sour-faced, Mrs. Larsen begrudgingly strode across the floor and stood with Noah behind a pew. It created a barrier between her and Violet. Obviously, Mrs. Larsen wasn't feeling the Christmas spirit.

Violet wasted no time and worked her way around the pew to get beside them. "Merry Christmas, Ma." She turned to Noah. "You, too, sweetheart."

The child lifted his arms toward Violet. "Sissy."

Mrs. Larsen strengthened her hold on the boy, and he whimpered and squirmed. "Your sister can't hold you right now, Noah," she snapped. "I've got you." She could barely keep her arms around him. He'd gotten so big that when he started wriggling, she almost dropped him.

"Oh, my." Gideon's ma wormed her way along the pew from the other direction and placed herself in front of Mrs. Larsen, yet spoke to the child. "You're such a big boy. Let me take you." She jutted her chin and looked directly at Mrs. Larsen. "You don't mind, do you Rose?"

"Course not." Mrs. Larsen handed him over.

His ma jostled Noah all the way down the row, then moved around the pew and came up on the other end next to Violet. "Your baby brother is one a the sweetest children I reckon has ever been born in this cove. But my, oh my, is he ever heavy. Can *you* take him for a spell?"

Gideon had always loved his ma—that was a given. But he'd gained a new kind of respect for her. This display of love for Violet would be something he'd remember forever.

Violet drew Noah close, and he clung to her.

"Sissy," he repeated, and rested his head on her shoulder.

"Merry Christmas, Noah." She stroked his head. "I love you."

"Rose?" Gideon's ma placed herself between Violet and her ma. "Violet and I have been cookin' since yesterday, an' I have a nice ham in the oven. We'd love to have your family join us for Christmas dinner."

His pa sauntered up beside her. "That's right." He nodded at Mr. Larsen. "We got plenty a food. Enough for all your boys, too."

Mrs. Larsen fidgeted with the collar on her coat, shaking her head and giving her husband the eye.

He scratched the back of his neck. "We'll hafta pass, but we 'preciate the offer. Rose has been cookin' herself. You know—old family recipes an' such for the holiday."

"That's right," Mrs. Larsen said. "We best be gettin' home." She headed straight for Violet. "C'mon, Noah. We gotta go." She held out her hands, but the child didn't budge. If anything, he held Violet tighter.

Mrs. Larsen huffed. "I said, we hafta go. Let go a your sister this minute." She pried him from Violet's grasp.

Noah wailed. The most heart-breaking sound Gideon had heard since the war. Making matters worse, Violet's eyes teared up.

Her happiness had been snuffed out.

Mrs. Larsen marched from the church with Noah thrown over her shoulder like a sack of potatoes. Her husband and the two boys obediently followed.

Violet clutched onto Gideon. "Look at him." She panted out breaths and sniffled. "Noah wants *me*."

The little boy's hands opened and closed as he reached back toward them, bawling. "Sissy!"

"Hush, Noah," Mrs. Larsen fussed and kept going.

Violet buried her face against Gideon's chest. "Take me home. Please?"

He nodded and led her out into the cold air.

* * *

Violet cuddled against Gideon in the wagon. His pa drove the horses extra slow along the road. Tiny flakes of snow danced around them and had already blanketed the ground in solid white.

Gideon's ma mumbled something under her breath that Violet couldn't discern. But she assumed it had to do with the way her own ma had behaved.

"We used to laugh together," Violet whispered. "My ma was happy. I miss that person. She ain't the same woman no more."

Gideon drew her closer to him. "Pay her no mind. If what your pa says is true, she's sick an' can't help how she behaves. Don't let it ruin your Christmas."

"That's right," his ma boldly said. "You was singin' so purty back there. I imagine the angels in heaven is lookin' forward to the day you join their chorus."

"Ma!" Gideon glared at her. "Don't be talkin' like that. I want her *here* singin' for us. I don't wanna think 'bout the other."

"It was a compliment, son." She shook her head, then smiled at Violet. "You didn't take no offense, did ya?"

"No'm. I'm glad you like how I sing." She twisted her fingers around each other. "I planned to wait till later to give Gideon this present, but I need sumthin' to lift my spirit again." She took hold of Gideon's hand. "Do you mind if I give it to you now?"

His eyes shifted back and forth between his folks and her. "You want to give it to me in front a my folks?"

"Uh-huh." She studied his curious expression. "What's wrong? You look like you swallowed a possum."

"Don't you reckon we should be more . . . *private*?"

The expression on his face tickled her, and it certainly lifted her spirits. "You silly man. I ain't gonna do nothin' embarrassin'." She lightly smacked his arm.

"Oh. I thought when you said you was gonna give me another gift when we were alone . . . well . . . you know." His cheeks were already red from the cold, but they turned an even deeper shade.

His pa cleared his throat. "Son, why don't you just let your wife say what's on her mind?"

His ma chuckled and waved a hand. "Go on, Violet. Gideon's gonna seal his yapper till you finish."

Violet sat up and turned sideways in the seat, so she could see everyone clearly. Mr. Myers pulled the team to a halt and shifted to face her.

The beauty that surrounded them took her breath. Evergreens had been frosted with puffy white snow. The sun shimmered on the meadow and reflected off the blanketed ground. Tiny crystals got caught in their hair and on their clothes, and alit on the backs of the horses. A hush had fallen over the valley.

Christmas peace wiped away her ma's harshness. "I love you all so much. I can't think of anywhere else I'd rather be than with you." She peered directly into Gideon's eyes. "But I think it's high time we share all this love with someone else. Someone real small who's gonna thrive in this lovin' family."

Gideon frowned. "Violet. We've talked 'bout this. You know your folks ain't gonna let you take Noah."

Violet stroked the backs of his hands. "I ain't talkin' 'bout Noah. I'm talkin' 'bout a little someone that no one will ever be able to take from us. Cuz he or *she* will be ours." She kept her eyes on his face, hoping for comprehension.

His frown melted away and conformed into the strangest expression imaginable. Her husband had had his share of odd expressions, but this topped it all. His eyes widened, then formed into slits, then his mouth dropped open, and he looked as if he might be sick.

"A baby?" He said the word as if it were foreign.

"Yep. I figger it'll come 'round the middle a July." His reaction wasn't at all what she'd expected. Why hadn't he whooped and hollered? "Gideon? Are you angry?"

"Huh?" He gaped at her. "Angry? Lordy, Violet. Nothin's ever made me happier. I just don't know what to do with myself. I'm gonna be a pa." He patted his pa's back. "Did you hear me? *I'm gonna be a pa!*"

His ma burst out crying. "I'll be a granny!" She took Violet's hand. "Scooch yourself over closer to Gideon. You're too near the edge a the wagon. Can't have you fallin' out!"

Mr. Myers wiped tears from his eyes. "Call me grampa. Best Christmas gift since the baby Jesus was born."

Mrs. Myers snuggled against her husband and the two chattered on and on about the coming baby.

Their happiness thrilled Violet, yet she focused on her husband. His reaction mattered the most. "You sure this didn't happen too soon for your likin'?"

"Course not. I knew you wanted a baby all along. You made that clear." He put his mouth to her ear. "'Specially on our weddin' night." He whispered the words, gave her a quick peck on the cheek, then leaned away from her, grinning.

She giggled. The joy of the season had returned two-fold.

Mr. Myers got the horses moving again and they headed home. A fine dinner awaited them. And since Violet was now eating for two, she'd take advantage and eat as much as she wanted.

Chapter 18

Lily had never seen anything like this. Brown paper lay strewn everywhere, along with brightly colored bows. Each of the children had gotten a stocking full of small trinkets and candy, as well as multiple wrapped gifts.

If her ma were there, she'd see this as a disgusting spectacle that spoiled the children and tainted the reason for the holiday.

Lily, however, viewed it as a blessed gift. The children appreciated each and every item and thanked their folks for the presents under the tree. The things in the stockings were attributed to Santa Claus, and he got his own thanks. They hollered up the chimney.

Arabelle pushed on the wheels of her chair and rolled over to Lily. "You're being very quiet. Are you all right?"

"I'm fine. *Truly.*" Lily emphasized the word to prove she meant it, and promised herself she'd never lie to her friends again about her wellbeing. Whether or not she felt like talking about it. "I'm just takin' it all in." She nodded toward Jenny. "Were you surprised at the gift she asked for?"

"Yes. But it warmed my heart. Of the three girls, Jenny has played with the dollhouse the most. She treasures every piece of furniture—especially since you made them pick up the pieces from the floor of their room." She let out a soft laugh. "Jenny enjoys rearranging the rooms, and now that her little mother doll has a wheelchair, she said she was going to place the furniture so the doll can easily move around it."

"The man who made the wheelchair, did a wonderful job. It had to be hard workin' with such small pieces."

"He's a fine craftsman. Arthur said he took extra care in making sure that the wheels would turn."

Lily fingered the soft lace collar on her blue dress. "I know another fine craftsman. I love what you did to my dress. The collar it had before irritated my skin. This one don't bother it at all."

"I assumed you hated that old collar. After all, you ripped it off. Another story you'd like to share?"

"Not today. I wanna enjoy Christmas with your family. An' maybe next year, my son will be part of it." She patted both hands on her lap, then stood. "I gotta get workin' on dinner. Wanna help?"

Arabelle cocked her head to one side and touched her hand to her chest. "Me? I don't cook."

"Ever peel potatoes?"

"Many years ago, but—"

"Don't try foolin' me into thinkin' you can't do anythin' with them hands." Again, Lily ran her fingers around the lacy collar. "I know better."

"But . . ."

Lily eyed her closely, then understood her hesitation. "I know. I'm the hired help an' it's part a my job. However, I think it might do you some good to learn a little 'bout keepin' up a kitchen an' fixin' meals. I might get ill someday, an' someone's gonna hafta step in. I've been teachin' the girls, but I reckon you don't want them knowin' more than you do. Right?"

"I suppose not."

Satisfied, Lily paraded into the kitchen and Arabelle followed.

The counters had been built too high for Arabelle to do much of anything on them. So Lily put the potatoes and knife on the kitchen table and Arabelle parked herself there.

Lily would have to speak to Mr. Jacobson about getting a carpenter to redesign the kitchen and make it more suitable for Arabelle. If all went as Lily hoped, one day, this lovely family would be able to care for itself. Maybe by then, Lily would not only have Noah, but perhaps she'd meet someone special and have a family of her own.

***

Caleb rubbed his hands together and his mouth watered. The meal spread out on the white linen smelled incredible. Ham. Turkey. Fresh-baked rolls. Sweet potatoes. Mashed potatoes with gravy. Corn pudding. Peas and carrots. And . . .

He licked his lips. Both pecan and pumpkin pie made by his beautiful wife, of course.

Thanksgiving at the hotel had been just as grand. Caleb never complained about a fine meal.

He glanced at Rebecca and his mood changed. He hated to admit it, but his ma was right about her. She'd gotten too thin. Her cheeks had sunken in somewhat, and the dress he'd bought her for Christmas hung loose at her shoulders. She'd worn it regardless, but it definitely needed to be altered.

She rarely ate much of anything at home, but surely, she'd eat *this* food.

They shared the table with not only little Avery and his ma, but also Mr. and Mrs. Iverson, the owners of the hotel. Other hotel guests and folks who didn't want to cook their own meals sat at three other tables. Happy chatter filled the dining hall.

"Let's not have the food get cold," his ma said. "Caleb, why don't you start, then pass it around?"

"Yes'm." He speared a piece of ham, put it on his plate, then gestured to a piece for Rebecca. "I can put one on *your* plate if you'd like."

She kept her hands folded on her lap. "I don't care for any, thank you."

"No ham?" Caleb hesitated, then passed the platter to Mrs. Iverson, who sat on the other side of Rebecca. "You'll eat some turkey, won't you Becca?"

"No meat. My stomach's a mite upset." She patted her belly. "Perhaps some potatoes without gravy."

Even without looking at her, Caleb felt his ma's eyes on them. He glanced her way and sure enough, she'd been watching. Her brows crinkled together in worry.

Caleb rested a hand on Rebecca's leg. "Sweetheart, you need to try to eat more than taters. Maybe some peas an' carrots, too?"

"All right. I'll try."

He scooped several spoonfuls of vegetables onto his plate as well as hers. Avery sat to his right in a highchair provided by the hotel. She readily ate whatever was set on her plate. His ma sat at the other side of the baby and made certain all her meat was cut into bite-size pieces.

The Iverson's talked to his ma, but he paid no mind to their conversation. He couldn't keep his eyes or attention off Rebecca.

She poked at the potatoes with the tip of her fork, then pushed several peas around the plate. Her face stayed expressionless, as if she'd died inside.

Caleb leaned back and reached over to this ma. "Can you keep an eye on Avery for a bit?" he whispered. "I'm gonna take Becca out an' have a talk."

"*Now*? In the middle a dinner?"

"She ain't eatin', Ma. Reckon now's the perfect time."

His ma slowly nodded. "Don't worry 'bout Avery. We'll be fine. Won't we?" She tickled under Avery's chin and prompted a giggle.

Caleb scooted his chair back, then reached for Rebecca. "Come with me a minute. All right?"

She gave a simple nod, and Caleb helped her to her feet.

He put an arm around her and led her from the dining hall. They'd not even taken two steps from the room, when her knees buckled and she went down.

Fortunately, he kept her from falling all the way to the floor. He scooped her into his arms and carried her to a chaise in the lobby, then gently set her down.

"Becca?" He sat beside her and cradled her against him. "What's happenin' to you?"

Tears seeped onto her cheeks, but she didn't make a sound. "I thought I was with child."

"What? Why didn't you tell me?"

She lay limply in his arms. "I wanted it to be a surprise. I went to Doc Garrison, just to be sure. I told him I hadn't had a flow in over a month. But . . ." She took several gasping breaths. "He told me there's no baby. He said I've gotten so thin that my body's not workin' right."

"Then you gotta start eatin'. It's the only way you'll get better." He stroked her cheek and tried to get her to look at him, but she kept her eyes focused downward. "You hear me? Eat an' it'll take care a everythin'."

"I can't. I get so depressed 'bout not conceivin', I don't want to eat. Food doesn't appeal to me anymore. I can't cook it, an' I can't eat it." She finally lifted her eyes. "Seems I'm my own worst enemy."

He was tempted to tell her how foolish she was being, but he knew it wouldn't help. Still, he had to do *something*. If she kept this up, he'd lose her.

"Do you still wanna move into the hotel?" He had no idea how he'd work it out, but he'd find a way. "Would that help?"

"No. I want to be near you. With winter here, you have to be on the farm to tend the animals. The only way we could live here, is if you found someone to take over for you. Maybe even *sell* the farm. We have to stay together. Could you do that?"

Sell the farm?

It was his life. The very thing that gave him purpose. Somehow, he had to stall her without making her believe he wouldn't do whatever it took to help her. After all, if he sold the farm, *he'd* die inside. "I doubt anyone would buy this time a year. Most folks are hunkered down for the winter. Maybe come spring."

She sadly nodded.

"Tell you what . . ." He gulped. "Why don't I ask Ma to come live with us till then? She can cook an' help tend Avery. It'll give you the chance to get your strength back."

Rebecca sat up. "Reckon she would? She's always said we need our own space."

He ran his fingers along her hair. "That's true, but she's been worried 'bout you. I think she'd come if we asked."

"I like the idea." Finally, she smiled. He hadn't seen one from her all day. "I've missed havin' her 'round. She an' I have always gotten on quite well."

"Good. Let's go ask her, an' I want you to give another try at eatin'." He placed his hands to her cheeks. "Will you do that for me?"

"Yes."

He kissed her lips, then her forehead, and helped her from the chaise. All the way back to the dining hall, he kept a firm hold on her.

Her obsession with bearing their child had to end. If it wasn't meant to be, they couldn't do anything about it.

Perhaps God had something else in mind.

Chapter 19

Violet turned sideways and smoothed her dress over her slightly rounded belly. She was well into her fifth month. "Look, Ma. Your grandchild is gettin' bigger."

Her dear mother-in-law set aside the washcloth she'd been using to scrub the counters and crossed the floor to Violet. "May I?" She gestured to the bulge.

"Course you can. I don't mind."

Mrs. Myers laid her hand on the spot. "Have you been feelin' it move some?"

"A bit. But not so much that Gideon can tell. He wants to feel it kick, but I ain't lookin' forward to that." She sighed. "I'm just glad this long winter is over."

Mrs. Myers chuckled. "You won't be sayin' that when you're in your ninth month an' it's hot as the blazes. Trust me, that'll be far more uncomfortable than a kickin' baby."

Violet rested her hand atop her mother-in-law's. "I'm tryin' to enjoy every part of my pregnancy. I like the eatin' part the best."

They both jumped when someone pounded on their door.

"What in heaven's name?" Mrs. Myers scurried across the room and opened the door wide. "Mr. Larsen?" His ashen face dimmed Violet's joy. "What's wrong?"

Violet rushed over to them. "Pa?" His eyes widened in panic and completely doused her happy mood. She tried to grab his arm, but he jerked away. "Don't touch me. I don't want you to take any chances."

"What are you talkin' 'bout? Come inside an' tell us what's goin' on."

"I can't. I gotta get back to Rose. But you . . ." He pointed a stern finger at Violet. "Stay as far away as you can. Best if you don't leave this house for a long spell. Hear me?"

Mrs. Myers gently pushed Violet behind her. "Someone's sick, ain't they?"

"Sick?" Violet looked from one scared face to another. "Is it Ma?"

Her pa nodded. "Yep. But that ain't all." He wiped sweat from his forehead. "Noah an' the other boys got it, too."

Violet clutched her chest. "What've they got, Pa?" She shut her eyes fearing the worst.

"The pox. Them *chicken* kind. You know the ones what make the skin look like a plucked bird. Rose an' the boys got blisters everywhere. Awfullest sight I ever seen."

Violet's knees weakened, so she grasped onto her mother-in-law's shoulder. "How'd they get 'em? They had to come from *some*where."

"The Hendersons went to Gatlinburg for supplies. They visited some a their kin folk while they was there an' figgered they musta brung the sickness back with them. They swear they didn't know anyone was sick, but shortly after they got home, the babies came down with it. They gave it to Noah an' he passed it on to your ma an' the boys."

Anger replaced fear. Violet leered at him. "He wouldn't a got 'em if you'd a kept him home where he belongs!" She yanked her coat from the wall. "I gotta go tend him. It's obvious *you* can't!"

Mrs. Myers grabbed hold of both of Violet's arms and stopped her. She peered deep into Violet's eyes. "You lost your senses? Them pox is highly contagious. You get 'em, and we could lose you *an'* the baby."

Violet's chin trembled, but she pushed down tears. She snapped her head toward the door and glared at her pa. "Why ain't *you* got 'em if they're so catchin'?"

"Cuz I had 'em when I was a boy. Once you get 'em, you don't get 'em again. Your sister had 'em when she was 'bout Noah's age. Your ma was carryin' you at the time. I kept Lily away till she got better. I didn't wanna risk losin' Rose. See . . . the pox is harder on grown folks than children. At your ma's age now . . ." His face scrunched up and Violet could tell that he, too, fought tears.

Knowing Noah and her brothers would likely be fine helped some, but the reality of her ma's situation struck deep. She couldn't be angry at her pa any longer. "You're sayin' . . . Ma could die?"

He didn't answer. His eyes shut and his head dropped low.

"What can we do, Buck?" Mrs. Myers asked.

He gradually lifted his head. "I need word sent to my other children. Lucas an' Lily should know 'bout their ma."

"I'll get Haywood to send telegrams. We got Lily's address, but where should we send word to your boy?"

"He's in Knoxville. Stayin' at the home a Captain Ableman's widow. With that much information, I reckon the law can find him an' give him the news."

"Yes." Mrs. Myers released a sad sigh. "That should do."

"Tell your husband I 'preciate the help. Now, I best go. Rose is runnin' a high fever." He looked straight at Violet. "Anythin' you want me to tell your ma?"

Violet put her back to him. So many thoughts tumbled through her mind, she didn't know what to say. Though she'd been feeling poorly about her ma in recent times, Violet couldn't comprehend the thought of never seeing her again.

She built up courage and faced him. "Tell her I love her an' always have. But Pa, you gotta promise me you'll take care a Noah. He's so little. An'—"

"He'll be fine. You best be sayin' some prayers for your brothers. They got it worse than him."

"Pa . . . don't you think we should tell Lily 'bout Noah?"

He cast a leery eye at Mrs. Myers, then returned his gaze to Violet. "She should know 'bout *all* her brothers."

Mrs. Myers put her arm around Violet. "Go on now, Buck. An' please, tell Rose we're keepin' her an' your boys in our prayers."

His head bobbed a couple times, then he ran off.

Violet latched onto her mother-in-law. "I'm so scared. I might a been mad at my ma for all her hatefulness, but I don't want her to die."

"Course you don't." Mrs. Myers tenderly rubbed Violet's back. "Tell you what. Let's go to the barn an' fetch the men. I gotta tell Haywood 'bout sendin' them telegrams, an' you can tell Gideon how you're feelin' 'bout what's happened. It'll make you feel better to share it with him."

"Have you ever had the pox? The chicken kind?"

"Yep. Haywood an' Gideon, too. Long time ago." Mrs. Myers lifted Violet's chin and stared into her eyes. "I'd go help your family if I wasn't so worried I'd come home an' pass on sumthin' to you. No one knows how the sickness travels, an' I don't wanna take a chance with you or my granbaby. You're too precious to me."

"I'm glad you can't get sick. The others neither. But my baby . . ." Violet protectively covered her belly. "I'm scared for my baby."

"Then you stay right here. I'll fetch Gideon an' bring him back. An' if it makes you feel more comfortable, for now, the two a you can stay in his old room 'stead a the weaner house. That way, I'll be nice an' close if you need me."

"You're the best ma ever." She kissed the dear woman's cheek. "Thank you."

While her mother-in-law shared the news with the men, Violet took a seat on the sofa and waited.

"I'll protect you best I can," she whispered and ran small circles over her unborn child with the tips of her fingers.

She shut her eyes.

God, help us all . . .

* * *

Lily grinned at the sound of Mr. Jacobson's clinking coffee cup. She hopped out of bed and flung her curtains open. Glorious spring sunshine covered her in a blanket of warmth.

The winter weather had been milder in Asheville than she'd expected. They had *some* snow, but not a great deal. Heavier snow had covered her beautiful mountains, but even it had started to vanish.

Soon, the roads would be clear enough to travel. Mr. Jacobson had promised to arrange for an honorable man to accompany her to the cove. Even though she'd told him that she was capable of making the trip alone, neither of the Jacobsons would hear of it. They insisted she have a companion.

She quickly dressed, strolled into the kitchen, and doctored her coffee. Humming, she took her seat at the table.

"You seem quite chipper this morning," Mr. Jacobson said. "Sleep well?"

"Yessir. Better every day." She sipped her coffee. "Spring has arrived an' I'm ready to get my life in order."

"Don't rush to trek over the mountain just yet. It can be very muddy in the spring."

"I don't care. Long as the driver can get the buggy there, that's all that matters. A little mud never hurt me."

She took another sip, then realized something was out of order. "Where's Levi?"

Mr. Jacobson chuckled. "He crawled in bed with us in the middle of the night. He's still curled up beside his mother."

Lily let out a happy sigh, brought about by thoughts of her own son. "That's so precious."

"Yes, it is." Mr. Jacobson eyed her over the rim of his cup. "Have I told you recently how much I appreciate what you've done for us?"

"Yep. Least a dozen times."

"Good. I don't want you to forget it." He stood and set his cup on the counter. "And since you've been so good to us, and the weather is becoming more favorable, I'll look into hiring the driver we spoke of . . ." He grinned at her. "As well as a carpenter to redesign this kitchen. I'm glad you suggested it."

Her heart danced. Soon, she'd see her son. "Thank you. For everythin'. Bringin' me here, makin' me part a your family, an' now, helpin' me get back to my son."

"It's the least we can do. Selfishly, I want the two of you to return to Asheville as soon as possible. I can't imagine our home without you."

"I can." She no longer had any doubts. "Y'all would do fine if I left for good. Since you're followin' through with my suggestion 'bout the kitchen, I reckon you'll see an even bigger change in Arabelle. She's decided she likes to cook, so you might not be able to get her outta the kitchen, once it's set just right."

His eyes lowered, but almost instantly lifted. They held a dreaminess about them, and he cast a soft, tender smile. "You told me she needed purpose. You couldn't have been more correct. She's become the woman I remembered. The one I fell in love with."

Lily pondered his remark. "But you never stopped lovin' her, did you? Even when she was havin' such a hard time?"

"Of course not. In many ways, my love grew. It made me realize what's truly important, and I can't imagine my life without her."

"I knew you two were special right from the start." Lily set her cup down and traced invisible patterns on the tabletop. "I hope I find someone as special. I thought I had once, but I was wrong."

"I have no doubt you will. As for being wrong, from my understanding, the heart doesn't lie. Sometimes circumstances get in the way and prevent people from following their feelings. However, I believe all things happen for a reason. Even something as horrid as Arabelle's accident. She and I can look back now and see the good that it's brought us. Including you. So don't give up, Lily. God has a bigger plan. Complicated as it might be. After all, He *is* God. He's allowed to be complicated."

As serious as he was being, his comment tickled her and she couldn't help but laugh. "For a man who hasn't gone to church in a great while, you sure seem to have a strong understandin' of the Lord."

"Not exactly. But fortunately, *He* understands *me*." He chuckled and nodded toward the door. "I'd better get to work, or I'll be late opening for business."

"I gotta get busy, too. I coulda sworn I heard Levi in there babblin' at his ma."

"Then I'll sneak out before he can miss me."

Mr. Jacobson inched out the door and was gone before Lily could blink.

She finished her coffee, then headed to Arabelle's room. Lily had barely gotten her friend dressed and in her wheelchair, when the front door opened.

"That's odd," Lily said.

Before she could go and see who'd come in, Mr. Jacobson appeared in the doorway of the bedroom.

"Forget sumthin'?" Relieved it was him, Lily grinned at the man.

"No." His typical smile was nowhere to be seen. "This came for you." He extended a piece of paper. "It's a telegram from the cove."

Lily stared at the thing, afraid to take it. "It's gotta be bad news. Just when things seemed to be fallin' into place. I don't wanna read it. You do it."

Arabelle rolled up beside her. "It's likely private, Lily."

"I don't care. Y'all know most everythin' 'bout me. Nothin's too private to share with the two a you." She waved her hand. "Go on, Mr. Jacobson. Read the thing."

He opened the telegram. "It was sent from Mr. Haywood Myers. I don't recall you mentioning anyone by that name."

"He's my sister's father-in-law." Lily's heart tripled its speed. *If sumthin's happened to Violet . . .* "What's it say?"

He quickly scanned it. "These are so impersonal."

Lily could scarcely breathe. "It's bad, ain't it?"

He lowered it from in front of his face. "Lily, your mother and brothers have chickenpox. Your mother's not doing well."

"My brothers?" She clutched her stomach, feeling sick herself. "Does it say which brothers?"

"No. It only refers to brothers. No specific names."

"Oh, God." Lily sat down hard on the edge of the bed. "Noah . . ."

"But he's your son. Wouldn't they have said . . .?"

"No." Lily covered her face with her hands. "My folks made everyone in the cove think he's theirs, so of course Mr. Myers would refer to him as my brother." She snapped fully upright. "I gotta go."

She flew from Arabelle's room into her own and dug out her

knapsack. She stuffed in personal items, then went to the kitchen and scanned for food to take on the trip.

Mr. Jacobson gripped her shoulder. "Lily. Slow down. I understand your urgency, but I need to hire a driver."

"I'll go myself. I ain't got time to wait."

"Yes, you do." He turned her to face him. "Have you ever had the chickenpox?"

"Yep. When I was real little. I can't get 'em again." She frantically looked around her, realizing the responsibilities she'd be leaving behind. She should already be cooking breakfast for the children and getting them ready for the day.

"Mr. Jacobson." She swallowed hard. "I know you count on me for many things, but my family needs me. Please understand."

Arabelle entered the room with Levi behind the wheelchair pretending to push it. "Arthur and I both understand, Lily. I'm sure I can speak for Arthur when I say that we want you to go."

He nodded. "But not alone. We've discussed this."

"Then find me a driver. Please?"

"I will. It shouldn't take long. I spoke to Hiram Baldwin a few weeks back about the possibility. He said he'd be happy to escort you."

"Hiram, huh?" Lily worked her lower lip with her teeth. "Is he old an' decrepit? I need someone strong who can manage the mountain roads, an' who doesn't mind sleepin' in the open air."

"He'll be fine. He's around thirty-five and quite fit. He's married with six children. His family needs the money."

Lily rubbed her aching chest. "He'll do. Thank you."

"You're welcome. Go on and get ready to leave, and I'll be back for you as soon as I can. I know you'll want to tell the children goodbye." He knelt next to Arabelle. "Will you be all right when Lily goes?"

"Yes. I discovered I'm capable of many things. And whatever I can't do myself, the girls will assist me."

Levi peeked out from behind the wheelchair. "I 'sist, too."

Mr. Jacobson knelt down, ruffled the boy's hair, then kissed Arabelle on the cheek. "As I said, I'll come back as soon as possible." He hurried out the door.

For some reason, the sound of the slamming door released Lily's dammed-up tears. She dropped to the floor and sobbed.

Arabelle moved beside her and lightly touched the top of her head. "Noah will be fine. He's big enough to fight off the illness."

Lily drew her knees to her chest and rocked back and forth. "I hate bein' so far away. I feel helpless."

"Mother?" Winnie crept into the room. "Why's Miss Larsen crying?"

"Her family is sick. Your father is hiring a driver to take her home."

Winnie knelt next to Lily. "You're leaving us?"

"Miss Larsen is leaving?" Jenny added her worried voice.

Lily wiped her eyes and tried to compose herself. She spotted Opal behind her sisters. Every face in the room looked dismally sad.

"I'm sorry," Lily said. "I love you all so much, and I'm proud of how you've worked so hard an' helped your ma. I swear you've all grown up in the short time I've been here. But I gotta go. I promise, I'll come back. I just don't know when."

The girls dropped onto the floor beside her. Numerous loving arms encircled her, and the children cried right along with her.

Lily had been happy about the idea of going home. She'd intended to go to her folks with strong resolve and reclaim her son. Then she'd planned to bring him back to Asheville with her and make a new life for them.

All that had changed. She feared what she might find in Cades Cove.

Losing Noah would completely break her.

Chapter 20

Gideon rolled onto his side and tenderly rubbed Violet's arm. "Sweetheart, you gotta stop cryin'. It's makin' you sick, an' I know it ain't good for the baby."

"But . . ." She sniffled and lay on her back. "I wanna do sumthin' to help my family, an' I can't. How long will I hafta stay inside? It can't hurt to go out an' enjoy some sunshine. Can it?"

"I don't know. There's a dozen or more folks sick in the cove. Them pox done spread like wildfire. For all we know, it might carry in the wind." He placed a soft kiss on her cheek. "I don't wanna take any chances." His hand glided downward and he lightly patted her belly. "It's best you stay in."

Strangely, she laughed. "Are you talkin' to me or the baby?"

When he realized what he'd said, he laughed along with her. "Both, I reckon. But *he* best be stayin' in *you* least another four months."

She coyly lowered her eyes.

Gideon stroked her face. "I'm glad I made you smile."

"Gideon?" His pa rapped on their bedroom door.

"Yeah, Pa?"

"I heard you talkin', so I knew you was awake. I need to talk to you." His voice held a sense of urgency.

"Sumthin' wrong?"

"Just get dressed an' come on out here."

Gideon flipped the covers off, then swung his leg around. He grabbed his crutch and hoisted himself up. "I don't like the way he sounded."

Violet also rose from the bed. "Me neither."

"Maybe you should stay in here. Pa asked for me, not us."

"Well, he didn't say I can't come out. 'Sides, if there's more bad news, I need to hear it."

They got their clothes on as fast as they could and headed into the living room. His ma sat on the sofa, wringing her hands. Not a good sign.

She waved to Violet, then patted the spot beside her. "Come sit, dear."

Violet wasted no time. "What happened? Is it my ma?"

Gideon's pa walked back and forth in front of the fireplace. He stopped and motioned Gideon to the sofa as well, so he took the place next to his wife. She latched onto his hand and held it tight.

"Go on an' tell 'em, Haywood." His ma's voice shook.

His pa set a chair in front of them and sat down hard. "Violet, your brother, Lucas, came home."

"He's here?" Violet didn't look pleased, but the scared expression on his pa's face told Gideon there was a lot more to it.

The man rubbed his temples. "Buck came by. I hardly recognized him. He's lost weight an' plumb worn out. He told me Lucas arrived a couple days ago. Since he was livin' in Knoxville, he got here quick once he got the telegram 'bout his ma."

He dropped his hands to his lap and nervously rubbed them up and down his legs. "Buck said the boy seemed genuinely upset 'bout his ma bein' so sick, an' even though Buck told him to stay away from her, he didn't. I 'magine he'll come down with them pox now."

"Lucas ain't never had no sense," Violet harshly muttered. "Pa will hafta tend him, too. It'll make him even more tuckered out."

Gideon squeezed her hand. "Don't get upset, all right?"

"Your pa won't hafta worry 'bout takin' care a him," his pa said. "There's a bigger problem than that. Lucas ran off. He hadn't shown signs of the pox yet, but he was exposed. It's only a matter a time."

"Well, good riddance." Violet sharply nodded. "But I hate that he'll likely pass it on to others. Lucas don't care if he hurts folks. That boy loves bringin' misery."

"There's more." Gideon's pa gulped hard. "Lucas took Noah with him."

Violet gasped. "What?" She violently shook her head. "No. Why would he do that?" Breathing hard, she clutched the front of her dress and twisted the material in her grasp. "Why?"

His ma put an arm around her. "You gotta keep calm, Violet. We'll figger this out."

"That's right," Gideon said. "Pa? Why'd he take the baby? An' why did Mr. Larsen let him?"

"He didn't. When he woke up this mornin', both a them was gone. Buck said Lucas had been fussin' 'bout Noah. Lucas blamed the boy for their ma bein' sick, an' said he was nothin' but trouble."

Violet jumped up from the sofa. "He's always hated Noah." She spun around and faced Gideon. "We gotta do sumthin'. We hafta go after 'em!"

"Go after 'em?" Gideon slowly got up and moved beside her. "We don't know where they went."

Violet paced around the room, shaking her head and mumbling. She'd stopped crying, but seeing her like this was much worse.

Gideon grabbed her by the waist and stopped her as gently as he could. "Violet. I know you're frettin' over Noah, but we hafta think this through. Let's sit down an' talk it out. Where do you reckon Lucas would take him?" He guided her back to the sofa.

His ma had gone into the kitchen and poured a glass of water. She handed it to Violet. "Take a nice, slow drink. It'll help."

Violet did as she asked, then held the glass with both of her hands and rested it on her lap. She faced Gideon's pa. "Do you know if my pa told Lucas where Lily is?"

He shrugged. "He said they was expectin' Lily any day. Them folks she's livin' with sent a telegram sayin' they'd hired a man to bring her here. Lucas probably knew Lily was comin'."

Violet huffed, then took another quick sip of her drink. "Lucas is the devil himself. If he knew she'd be arrivin', he took Noah so she couldn't see him. How can he be so hateful?" Her head whipped around toward Gideon. "There's only one person Lucas despises more than Noah."

"Who?"

She glanced at his folks, then looked straight at him. "Caleb," she whispered.

"Who's Caleb?" his ma asked.

Gideon searched Violet's face, needing permission to answer the question.

Violet gazed upward, then let out a long breath. "We best tell 'em. The way things is happenin' 'round here, nothin' will make sense 'less they know the whole truth."

His ma returned to the sofa. "Sounds like sumthin' I best hear sittin' down."

Violet took hold of her hand. "Ma? Noah ain't my brother, he's my nephew. He's Lily's son."

Gideon kept his eyes on his ma to see her reaction. There was no gasp—no remark. Just a simple expressionless nod.

His pa cleared his throat. "Hmm . . ." He rubbed his chin, then let out another *hmm*.

Gideon looked from one to the other. "Ain't neither a you gonna say more than, hmm?"

His pa opened his mouth, but nothing came out.

"What I reckon your pa is tryin' to say," his ma said. "Is that we're a mite surprised by this revelation, yet it kinda makes sense."

Violet's head tipped to the side. "How?"

"Haywood an' me's talked over this before. The way Rose has treated that boy ain't right. She was all puffed up an' proud right after he was born, then soon after, she always passed him off to you. I didn't wanna say nothin', but sometimes I seen her look at Noah as if she detested him. I figgered she was just gettin' on in years, an' he was wearin' her down." His ma's eyes shifted to her lap. "I'd give anythin' to have my other two boys in my arms again. It bothered me the way Rose paid Noah no mind. What kind a lovin' ma would do that?"

Violet caressed the back of his ma's hand. "My ma used to be lovin'. But she never seemed to have any genuine good feelin's for Noah. No matter how angry she was at Lily for havin' a baby 'thout bein' married, Noah was still her blood. Her grandson. I doubt she could see beyond how he came into the world." Violet gasped and held a hand to her heart. "Lily's comin' home. What'll she do when Noah ain't here?"

Her frightened eyes tore at Gideon's insides.

His pa scooted his chair closer. "Do you know where to find Noah's pa?"

Gideon's ma sat taller. "That's good thinkin', Haywood. I assume the Caleb you mentioned is the boy's pa. Maybe Lucas done took the child to *him*."

Violet's eyes widened much larger. "But that's all the way in Waynesville. Three day's ride from here. An' Noah's sick. Without proper care, he could die." Tears trickled down her cheeks. "That's probably what Lucas wants." Her eyes shut tight, her face puckered, and she clenched her fists. "I hate him."

"Sweetheart . . ." Gideon's ma stroked Violet's hair. "Hate will tear you up inside. I understand how upset you are, but don't hate."

Violet's eyes gradually opened and she stared straight ahead. "I know what you're sayin', but if Noah dies, I won't ever forgive Lucas." She turned sharply toward Gideon. "You gotta go after him. Ride Stardust as fast as you can to Waynesville. An' if the good Lord's willin', maybe you'll find 'em."

Gideon could tell she was doing all she could to keep from bawling. Violet had never cared to show such strong emotion in front of his folks. But how could he help her?

He leaned back into the sofa cushions, wishing he could sink into the floor. He'd do anything to make his wife happy, except . . .

"I can't ride, Violet. You know that."

"I don't know any such thing. You *won't* ride, but you can."

"Um . . ." His ma frowned and patted Violet's arm. "Have you forgotten his leg?"

"Course not. But he's the only one that can do this. I'd go if I could." She pleaded with her eyes. "Gideon, you know how much that boy means to me. Please? Do this for me."

He grabbed his crutch and stood. His stomach roiled and he was almost certain he was going to be sick. He wandered toward an open window and stuck his head outside so he could breathe in the fresh air.

If he went to Waynesville, not only would he have to ride hard and fast, he'd have to spend several nights in the woods. It was likely there'd be wild animals about. He was a decent shot and could defend himself, but he didn't like being anywhere alone after dark.

Even a man with *two* good legs took a risk traveling by himself.

"Gideon?" Violet came up behind him. "I know you can ride."

His ma bustled over and joined them. "Violet, dear, you're askin' too much. Yes, my son can do a great deal, but there's limitations."

"Anna." Gideon's pa took his ma by the arm and led her to the side of the room. "Let *them* work this out."

Gideon inhaled deeply a final time, then pulled his head inside and faced Violet. "I'm scared. I know I'm a grown man, but this terrifies me."

"I understand." She stood tall and rapidly brushed tears from her cheeks. "But will you at least try sumthin' for me?"

If she truly understood, then maybe she wouldn't push him to ride. "I s'pose."

Violet took his hand. "With things the way they are, I'm not gonna be afraid to go outside to the barn. Far as I know, no one sick has come 'round here. So, come with me."

"Wait." His ma took a step toward them, but was stopped by his pa.

"I said, let them work it out, Anna."

She huffed, but stayed put.

Gideon went outside with Violet. She headed to the barn, and as he feared, she went straight to the mare's stall.

"Violet, I said I'm afraid. Don't that mean nothin' to you?"

She framed his face with her hands. "Course it does. I'm scared, too, but I'm not afraid to have you do this. You've feared many things since you came home 'thout that leg. You might still be layin' on your bed in the middle a the livin' room if I hadn't gotten you off your tail. I showed you, you can do things. An' as you know, you do some things I wish you wouldn't—like choppin' them logs." She stepped closer. "All I want is for you to climb up on Stardust's back an' see how it feels. Just . . . *try*."

She jerked her head toward the stall, then opened the latched gate and walked to the horse. Stardust whinnied as soon as Violet got close.

"That's my girl." Violet rubbed her nose and continued on down her back. "Let's get your saddle on. You ready to run?"

"Run?" Gideon's throat tightened. "Can't we start with walkin'?"

"Course you can. But it's senseless for you to go at all, if you ain't willin' to run. Noah's life's on the line. Don't you see?" She placed the saddle, then proficiently secured the straps. "C'mon, Gideon. Put your foot in the stirrup an' swing yourself up. I'll hold your crutch for you."

He remembered a time when he'd loved this. Being in the barn, smelling the fresh straw, and anticipating a good ride. He used to push his horse into a gallop anytime they were in an open field. He'd loved the sensation. Probably the closest thing to flying he'd ever experienced.

He inched toward the animal. If it were *his* son out there in the woods with a crazed uncle, he wouldn't have a second thought about getting on Stardust's back. They'd already be well on their way. So why was this any different? Noah was a helpless toddler, not to mention, *kin*.

He handed Violet the crutch, placed his foot securely in the stirrup, grabbed the horn, and hoisted himself up. Violet assisted with a hand to his rear, followed by a smile and a nod.

The encouraging gestures didn't help. He'd forgotten how high off the ground it was on the back of a horse, and Stardust was by no means small.

"Look at you, Gideon." Violet had stopped crying and beamed. "You did it."

"But we ain't movin'." He took several deep breaths and gazed at his beautiful wife. "Even so, I'll try."

"Thank you."

He leaned forward and grabbed the reins. Violet opened the stall gate wide and he eased the horse out.

"Remember, Gideon . . ." Violet kept pace beside them. "Squeeze your thighs together an' that'll keep you upright. You got your balance?"

They exited the barn. "Reckon so. I ain't fallen yet."

"Good. Now, click to her an' give her side a little nudge with your foot."

He shut his eyes and did as she asked.

Please keep me on here.

Stardust trotted a short distance down the road. Gideon teetered slightly, but capably turned her around and went back to the barn.

Violet took hold of the reins and brought Stardust to a halt.

Frowning, Gideon dismounted and took his crutch from Violet.

She stared at him. "Why do you look like that? I thought you did quite well."

He slowly bobbed his head. "Yep, I did. It's the very reason I'm frownin'. I ain't got no excuse not to go. Scared as I am, I think I can do this."

She hugged him so hard, he nearly toppled. "I knew you could!"

"Ma ain't gonna like it, but like Pa said, this was between us." He kept his eyes on his wife, wishing he didn't have to leave her, but knew there was no other choice. He memorized every curve of her face, then kissed her long and deep. "I love you. I'll search high an' low for Noah. An' I'll do all I can to bring him home."

"Thank you." She returned another kiss. "We best be packin' for your trip." She circled his waist with her arm, and they headed to the cabin.

Once he told his ma their plans, she'd be hard to handle. But he figured his pa could calm her down. After losing two boys, Gideon knew his ma didn't want to chance losing a third. He also believed that Noah wouldn't survive if someone didn't go looking for him.

He chose to put a helpless child ahead of his fears.

It was the right thing to do.

Chapter 21

One more night in the woods, then a half-day's ride would get Lily home. Until she knew what faced her, her heart wouldn't rest. It had been nearly impossible to sleep. Of course, Hiram's loud snoring didn't help.

They'd chosen a nice clearing to make camp for the night. Hiram went off to gather wood for the fire, and Lily spent her time making certain there were no rocks on the ground where she planned to make her bed. She'd tried sleeping in the buggy the first night, but found it horribly uncomfortable. The ground was more accommodating.

Sticks snapped not far from her.

Lily lifted her head to find Hiram pushing his way through some dense trees. His arms were loaded down with an assortment of wood. Mostly small broken limbs.

He set them on the ground. "We won't have any trouble stayin' warm t'night. Plenty a dry wood 'round here."

Before he'd left, he'd cleared a small area that he'd encircled with rocks. He stacked the wood in a pyramid shape and pushed in some kindling. "You said you grew up where we're headed. Ain't that right?"

He'd been more talkative than any driver Lily had previously traveled with. He was kind as he could be, but she didn't feel like talking. Even so, she couldn't be rude. Especially to someone as nice as Hiram. "Yep. I lived in Cades Cove most all my life."

He lit the fire, then sat on his rump and poked at it with a stick till it brightly flamed. "It's beautiful in these mountains. Peaceful, too."

Lily spread a blanket on her cleared spot and sat down. "Ain't you ever traveled in the Smokies?"

"Not much. Served my time in the war, but fought mostly farther south. I was one a the lucky ones who got to come home to my family. Good thing, too. Can't imagine Gloria handlin' our children alone."

Shortly after they'd first met, he'd told Lily all about his wife and six kids. If he asked her to repeat their names, Lily would fail miserably. She couldn't focus on anything but her own situation. She'd given him every indication that she'd been listening to all he'd had to say, but honestly, she'd scarcely heard a word. It might've been wrong to behave that way, but she couldn't help herself.

She lay back and stared upward at the darkening sky. Massive trees framed her view. "I'm sure your wife is missin' you right now."

"Reckon so. But she knows I'm comin' back. Nothin' like what she went through those years I was fightin'." He threw more wood on the fire. "You hungry? You ain't eaten hardly anythin'."

"I'm fine. I don't feel like eatin'." She positioned another blanket on top of herself and rolled onto her side. "I'm gonna try an' sleep. Maybe then, mornin' will come faster, so I can get home."

"That's a fine idea. I know you're frettin'. Folks in Asheville is prayin' for us, an' for your family, too. I hope you'll find them well when we get there."

"Thank you." As long as Noah was all right, Lily believed she could cope with anything.

"I'll try an' be quiet. The fire should keep the critters away. Hope you can sleep some."

Lily shut her eyes and listened to the fire crackle and the distant sound of owls and other skittering nighttime creatures. She never worried over much of anything in her mountains. Everything came second-nature to her here.

God, please keep Noah in your lovin' care.

Worn out and weary, she managed to drift into dreams.

* * *

Lily was ready for this trip to be over. Hiram had managed the small buggy well, and had it not been for the dire situation, she would've treasured the time in her beloved mountains. Yet urgency pushed her inwardly to get home and kept her from enjoying anything.

The two horses ably pulled the buggy, and they arrived in Cades Cove several hours sooner than Lily had expected. That suited her better than fine.

She guided Hiram along the dirt road to her folks' cabin. As they came nearer, nervous excitement filled her belly. She came close to jumping from the buggy and running the rest of the way, but forced herself to remain in the seat. She took the time to prepare her mind for whatever they might find.

They passed the wheat fields. The winter wheat crop looked healthy and would be ready for harvest in a few more weeks. The farm seemed to be thriving, though she saw a few things that needed tending.

Likely her pa had been unable, since he'd been caring for her ma and the boys.

She pointed to the cabin. "That's my home." Smoke billowed from the chimney.

Hiram steered the team close, then pulled them to a stop. "I'll wait here, while you look in on your family."

"You said you've had the pox. You're sure 'bout that, ain't you?"

"Yep. But I figgered you'd wanna see your family alone. Not with some stranger."

She patted his arm. "Thank you. Once I know whether or not I'll hafta stay for a while, you can make your plans to go back home."

"I ain't in no hurry, but Gloria is expectin' me within the week."

Lily nodded, then stepped down to the ground. She closed her eyes for a brief moment, then reopened them and took everything in. Her surroundings felt strangely foreign and familiar at the same time. Her heart continued to relentlessly pound.

She took slow deliberate steps to the front door. Her hand shook as she opened it.

"Pa?" The word barely squeaked out.

The foul odor in the air took her breath. She placed a hand over her mouth, then went to the kitchen window and opened it.

"Pa?"

Utter silence.

She forced her feet to move and headed toward her folks' bedroom.

A soft moan came from within.

The door stood ajar, so she gave it a small push and peeked inside. Her pa was sitting in the rocking chair beside the bed. His head was bent low and his chest steadily rose and fell.

He looked like a ghost of himself.

When she turned toward the bed, the sight there was far worse. Her ma's blistered face was unrecognizable. Her matted hair lay strewn about the pillow, and her pock-covered hands were folded atop her Bible, which rested on the blankets covering her stomach.

Lily crept into the room. As she neared her ma, she heard faint wheezing. It sounded as if her lungs had filled with fluid.

Lung fever.

Not good at all.

"Pa," Lily whispered. "I'm home."

The man's head popped up. "Lily?" He put his lone hand to his heart. His eyes filled with tears. "My Lily."

He tried to stand, but his legs wavered.

Lily grabbed hold of his arm and helped him to his feet. He held her close and cried.

"It's gonna be fine now, Pa. I'm home. I'll stay an' help as long as you need me."

He separated from her and motioned to the living room. "We hafta talk."

She understood. There was a lot that had to be said.

He took a few steps, but seemed so unsteady that she chose to hold onto him as they walked.

He glanced behind him at her ma before he shut the bedroom door. When they got to the sofa, they sat side by side.

In an odd way, it felt as if she'd never left.

"Pa, I understand you wantin' to talk an' all, but I wanna look in on the boys first. I gotta see that they're all right."

He grasped her hand, surprisingly hard. "Stay here with me, Lily. There's things you gotta know."

Her heart thumped harder than ever. "What is it? Is it my baby?" Tears stung her eyes, and her throat closed up.

Her pa stared at her with fear-filled eyes. "Lucas was here. He came home soon as I sent him word 'bout your ma."

"What did he do, Pa?" Panic had her trembling.

"He . . . He ran off with Noah."

Lily jumped to her feet.

Her pa grabbed at her, but she jerked free.

"Lily, there's more you need to know!"

She didn't want to hear any more from her pa. Noah couldn't be gone. He had to be here. She hurried to her old bedroom.

Empty.

She raced up the stairs to the loft.

"Lily?" Isaac sat up in bed and reached out to her.

She ran to him and held him as close as she could. "I've missed you so much." She couldn't hold back her tears any longer. "Oh, my poor boy. You're burnin' up." She stroked his damp head and studied the red sores on his face and arms.

"I'm better than I was, but I itch sumthin' awful." He scratched at one of the spots on his arm. "These things is all over me."

"Don't scratch. I know it's hard, but it'll only make it worse. I can fix up some medicine that'll help."

Horace moaned in the bed beside Isaac.

Isaac pointed at him. "He's a bigger baby than me. All he does is moan an' groan." Isaac's face scrunched up. "Did Pa tell you 'bout Noah?"

She nodded. "I'm gonna find him. Somehow."

Isaac's chin quivered. "Lucas is the meanest person I ever knowed. I tried to stop him. I heard him get up in the night an' saw some light downstairs. So I went to see what was happenin'. He told me to get back in bed. He was holdin' Noah so tight he was cryin'."

Lily felt like screaming, but she didn't want to upset Isaac further. "Then what happened?"

"He said he was takin' Noah where he belongs." Isaac sniffled. "Shouldn't he be here with us? He's my brother. I was gonna teach him how to play marbles."

"Shh . . ." She hugged him and rocked back and forth. "You'll get the chance. I promise." She stood and helped him lay back down, then covered him up real good. "Rest now. I'll be back soon with some medicine for them sores. I love you, Isaac."

"I love you, too, Lily." He sucked in several quick breaths. "Don't leave again. We need you here."

"I'll only leave to find Noah, then we'll both come home. All right?"

He nodded and sniffed, then burrowed his head into his pillow.

Lily hurried back down to her pa and sat on the sofa beside him. Her heart told her where she had to go.

"Pa, I gotta go to Waynesville. I reckon Lucas took Noah to Caleb."

The man's head bobbed. "That's what I figgered. It's the only place what makes sense. But Lucas has taken more than the child there. He's carried the pox with him. Anyone he comes in contact with is likely to catch it. Damn that boy for bein' so hateful."

"If my son dies, I swear I'll turn Lucas over to the authorities. He can rot in prison for all I care. He'd have two murders to answer to."

Her pa's shoulders slumped low. "I thought I raised that boy decent, but I was wrong." He blinked ever-so-slowly. "Lily, your ma's dyin'. Ain't nothin' can be done for her. Our family is fallin' apart, an' I don't know how to fix it."

Lily cuddled into his shoulder and wrapped an arm around his middle. She'd smelled death when she'd entered the cabin, so his words didn't surprise her. "I can make medicine for the boys that'll help with the itchin', but then I gotta go. I hafta find Noah, or I swear I'll go mad."

He stroked her hair. "Can you ever forgive me for sendin' you away?"

She lifted her head and met his gaze. "I will if you let me be his ma from now on."

He started to shake his head, but then he looked away and nodded. "Them boys upstairs will need a ma, too." A loud cry erupted from him. "What'll I do 'thout Rose?"

Her strong pa had become weak and defeated. The last time Lily had seen him this way, he was drunk on moonshine. "I'll come back an' do whatever I can to help. I know Violet will, too." She grabbed her pa's hand. "How is she Pa? She ain't sick, is she?"

"No. I made her stay away. She's with child. I couldn't risk her an' the baby."

Lily rapidly nodded. "She told me in a letter. I wanna see her, but I know it ain't a good idea. Not with me comin' in here an' all."

"That's right. Keep your distance from her. It's for the best. But, Lily . . .?"

"Yes, Pa?"

"You should go in an' make peace with your ma. She ain't been right for a while now, but there are days when she's aware. Don't let her die 'thout forgivin' her. You both need it said."

Lily sat upright and gazed into the firelight. "Let me gather the white oak for the medicine first. It'll help me put my mind right so I can talk to her an' say what's important."

He stood. "Fine. I'm goin' back to her now. Don't know how much longer she has."

"Did Lucas make his peace with her?"

He shook his head. "No one had peace while he was here. Your ma called him the devil an' made him stay away from her. It only made him angrier." He wandered to the bedroom and went in.

Lily returned to Hiram and let him know they'd be staying for only a few hours, then they'd be heading to Waynesville.

Lily despised her brother more than she imagined she could. He took a sick, innocent child on the run, not caring what happened to him. Noah didn't deserve to be put in the middle of Lucas's disdain for her and Caleb.

Lily's love for Noah would push her on until she found him. Alive or dead.

Chapter 22

Lily boiled some leaves and bark from a white oak tree. Normally, the leaves wouldn't be budded out quite yet, but she was fortunate enough to have found some. Once they'd steeped together with the bark long enough, she dipped a cloth into the water, then dabbed it on her brother's sores.

"Now remember . . ." She looked from Isaac to Horace. "Don't scratch. I'll leave some a this with Pa, so when you need more, let him know."

"Thank you, Lily," Horace muttered. "It's helpin'. Nothin' else has done any good."

"Them sores gotta dry up, so don't get 'em too wet. But a little wet is better than scratchin'."

She smoothed her hand over Horace's head. "I think you're gettin' better. Some a your sores have already formed scabs, but you gotta leave 'em alone. I reckon the worst of your sickness is over."

"Mine, too?" Isaac asked.

"Yep." She smiled. "You two look after each other. I'm goin' to find your brother, then I'll be home."

"For good?" Horace asked.

"Yep." She sat on his bed. "You both know that Ma's real bad off, don't you?"

"Uh-huh." Horace frowned. "We can hear Pa cryin' sometimes."

Isaac reached out to Lily. "Is she goin' off to Heaven soon?"

"Likely." Lily squeezed his hand. "But one day, we'll see her again. An' she won't be sick anymore."

Isaac's mouth twitched from side to side. "Will she be nice in Heaven?"

"*Everyone's* nice in Heaven," Horace said, before Lily could answer.

"That's right," Lily said. "Our ma will be the ma we remember." She stood and walked toward the stairs. "I love you both."

She traipsed down the stairs, knowing this next goodbye wouldn't be so easy. Her brothers were taking their ma's condition better than expected, but maybe they viewed it as a change for the better. None of them wanted her to hurt anymore. Or be hurt by her.

When she walked into her folks' bedroom, her pa got up from the rocker and motioned for her to take it.

The last time she'd sat in that chair, she'd been feeding Noah. The thought wrenched her heart.

Though her motherly instincts told her to leave as soon as possible to find her son, as her pa had said, she needed to make peace with her ma. If the woman was going to pass from this world, Lily wouldn't have another opportunity to set things right.

Her pa left the room and shut the door behind him.

"Buck?" her ma muttered.

Lily could scarcely bear to look at her ma's pocked face, but it was her raspy breath that pained Lily. Her ma struggled for every bit of air that passed her lips. Her rasps were followed by an awful gurgling sound.

"Pa's gone out." Lily scooted the rocker close to the bed, doing all she could to disregard the rank smell. "It's Lily, Ma. I've come home."

Her ma's head turned slightly and her half-shut eyes met Lily's. "Lily? Is that really you?" More gurgles, then a cough. Her ma licked her dry lips.

"Let me get you some water." Lily started to rise, but her ma lifted a hand. It shook in midair.

"No. I ain't thirsty."

Lily settled back in the chair. "Is there anythin' I can do for you?"

Her ma wheezed out several breaths. "Forgive me."

"I already have, Ma. I know you was tryin' to do what's best for me. I know I let you down, but I ain't a bad person."

"I know." She craned her neck and moaned. "Can you pull me up higher . . . on my pillow?"

"Course I can." Lily bent over her ma and reached under her arms. She used every ounce of strength she had to lift her, then readjusted the pillows and eased her ma back against them. The heat coming from the woman's body felt like fire.

Lily repositioned her Bible under her hands and straightened her blankets. She then sat back down in the rocker. "Better?"

"Yes." She seemed to be trying to open her eyes wider, but they wouldn't lift. Her ma had no strength whatsoever. "There's things you gotta know." Her words sounded like they were filled with bubbles.

"Ma, it's too hard for you to talk."

"I gotta." She swallowed hard, then took several short breaths. "I shouldn't a sent you to Helen. She . . ." More breaths. "She never forgave me for Buck."

"What's Aunt Helen got to do with Pa? Other than her fussin' 'bout how worthless he is."

"She was . . . in love with him. But he wanted . . . me." What looked like an attempt at a smile twitched her ma's lips. "Helen was jealous. Reckon she hated me for . . . for . . ." Her eyes closed completely.

"For marryin' him, Ma?"

Her head slightly bobbed.

"So," Lily said, "she married Uncle Stuart, an' she's been bitter ever since."

Her ma lifted a single finger. "My Lily. Such a smart girl." Her words were barely a whisper.

"Ma, please get some rest. I'm not angry 'bout you sendin' me there. I learned a lot 'bout myself." She took her ma's hand. "You was a good ma."

Her ma's lips moved, but Lily couldn't hear her, so she put her ear close to the woman's mouth. "Say it again, Ma."

"Take care a my boys."

Once again, tears pooled in Lily's eyes. Every ounce of anger she'd felt for her ma vanished. She intended to hold onto the memories of the woman she'd been long ago.

"Don't worry 'bout your boys, Ma. I'll love an' care for 'em till the day I die."

Lily could tell her ma had something else to say, so she bent near again.

The woman's hot breath covered Lily's ear. "Don't. Let. Lucas. Hurt. Noah."

Lily grasped onto her and cried. "I won't, Ma." Her ma lay limp in her arms, barely breathing, as if her final words were taking the remainder of her life.

Lily gently laid her down, then wiped away tears and crept from the room.

Her pa got up from the sofa the minute she came out. "Did you say your peace?"

"Yessir. Ma did, too."

"That's good." He stared at the floor and rubbed his forehead. "She tell you 'bout Helen?"

"She said Aunt Helen was in love with you. Is that true?"

"Yep. As the older sister, Helen shoulda been the first to marry. But I never had my sights on her. They was always on your ma. When I rejected Helen, she was determined to find her a *better man*—as she put it. One with money an' status."

Lily realized there was a great deal she didn't know about her folks. If she'd known this long ago, she would've understood Aunt Helen's hatefulness. Still . . .

"Pa? Why'd she act so ugly to *me*? I didn't do her wrong. Least, not till I embarrassed her when the truth 'bout me came out."

Her pa moved nearer. "Helen had no business actin' as she did. Even when she learned you'd birthed a child." He nervously licked his lips. "I don't like to talk 'bout this, cuz I don't feel it's right speakin' a such things. 'Specially with my daughter. But you're a grown woman an' you need to know the truth." He rubbed his chin, hesitating.

Lily remained silent, wondering what could be so bad.

He cleared his throat. "When Helen met Stuart Clark, she threw herself at him. She told Rose she'd found the finest man in the country, an' she'd do anythin' it took to hold onto him. She gave herself to him, then told him she was with child, so he'd marry her."

Lily gasped. "If that's so, she had no right to judge me for what I done. Her actions were much worse."

"That they were. To this day, I don't know how she convinced him she hadn't lied. Since the woman is barren, she musta come up with one helluva story."

"You an' Ma always said we lie to protect those we love. Aunt Helen did just that. She loves herself more than anyone."

Her pa hung his head. "But look where lyin' got us."

"Oh, Pa. How could you a known all this would happen? You didn't mean to hurt me an' Noah."

"That's right. But I did, an' now I hafta live with the consequences." He stood tall. "You best be goin' to find that boy. You got plenty a daylight left to get a good distance. Your driver watered the horses an' let 'em graze for a spell. They should be ready to travel."

Lily pulled him into an embrace. "I love you, Pa. An' I swear, I truly do forgive you. I appreciate you tellin' me the truth." She tightened her hold. "I hope I won't be long. Meanwhile, you best take care a yourself, an' please tell Violet I'll see her soon."

"I will." He patted her on the back. "Time's a wastin'. Go on now."

Lily kissed his cheek, then sped from the cabin.

* * *

Thank goodness spring had come. Rebecca disliked the cold winters.

She peered out the kitchen window. Though she couldn't see it from here, the silly swing beckoned her. Why she loved it so much, she wasn't certain. Perhaps it was because it took her back to a time when she was genuinely happy, and both Henry boys were alive.

She'd tried hard to let go of Abraham's memory, but hadn't done so well. Loving him had been easy, and she'd never questioned his love for her. It had been evident in every action—every look he'd given her.

Quite the opposite with Caleb.

Rebecca continued to have doubts about *his* feelings for her. Even though their relationship had improved since that day in the cemetery when he'd swore he wanted to start over again and stop wallowing over Abraham's death. Caleb had taken it so hard. She knew he loved his brother, but there was more to it. Likely because the two had disagreed on the war and had served on opposite sides. They'd not gotten the chance to come to terms with their disagreements. Once Abraham died, nothing could be done to set things right.

Yes, things had gotten better between Caleb and *her*, but there were times she'd see him gazing off as if he were somewhere else. Perhaps he *wanted* to be.

Along with her inability to conceive, she believed it was these kinds of thoughts that ruined her appetite and made her so thin.

Her mother-in-law had stayed with them up until two weeks ago. She'd been a great help through the winter, yet Rebecca was glad to see her leave. Not so much for herself and the need for privacy, but Rebecca knew Mrs. Henry would be happier by herself at the hotel. She'd become quite an independent woman who enjoyed setting her own schedule.

Rebecca hated the thought of being alone. But sometimes, even when Caleb was by her side, she felt exactly that way.

"I must truly be crazy," she mumbled.

"Pa!"

Avery's shout brought Rebecca out of her thoughts. Her daughter had been napping. Whenever she woke, she never cried out for Rebecca. She always called for Caleb. Their bond was undeniable.

Rebecca hurried to her room and lifted her from the bed. "Your pa's in the barn. One of our cows is havin' a baby, an' your pa's helpin'."

Avery rubbed her still-sleepy eyes. "Baby cow?"

"Yes. They're called calves. When it comes, I'm sure your pa will let us know. Then we can go see it. All right?"

Avery wriggled from her arms and went to her toy box. She picked up her stuffed cow and toddled back to Rebecca. "Moo Cow."

"That's right. That's your Moo Cow."

In a little over a month, her daughter would be two. Hard to believe so much time had passed.

A heavy-handed knock on the front door startled Rebecca and changed Avery's happy smile to a fearful frown.

"Caleb!" The harsh sound of a man's voice didn't help matters. "Caleb! Open this door!"

Rebecca scooped up her crying child. "Hush, baby."

Endless knocks became heavy thuds. Whoever was at the door obviously didn't intend to leave anytime soon.

Rebecca's heart raced. She didn't know whether to answer the door or flee out the back and fetch Caleb.

"Sweetheart." She set Avery back on the bed. "I need to go see who's out there. I'll just peek out the window, but I want you to sit right here an' wait for me. All right?"

Avery reached out. Rebecca couldn't expect her to understand.

"It's okay." She smoothed her hand over the child's head. "No one's goin' to hurt you. Hold tight onto Moo Cow, an' I'll be right back." Rebecca kissed her forehead, then left her room and crept toward the living room window.

She pressed her body against the wall and inched over until she could see the front porch. A red-haired man stood there holding a child who was poorly draped in a ragged blanket. Its bare feet hung out the bottom.

The man's eyes were half shut, and his brow was beaded with sweat. "Caleb!" He pounded again and again. "Open up!"

"Oh, my." Rebecca tried to still her racing heart.

Though he looked a great deal more unkempt, there was no mistaking who the man was. But why had Lucas Larsen come back? The child he was holding brought even more questions to Rebecca's mind.

Lucas's incessant yelling and door-ramming upset the child and it let out a squall.

Rebecca ached for the poor baby. The weather had warmed, yet the child was severely underdressed.

She swallowed hard and swung the door open.

Lucas breathed heavy and fast. "'Bout time." He stumbled inside and nearly dropped the baby.

Rebecca grabbed the child and shut the door. "What's this all 'bout?" She built up her courage and challenged him. "Tell me this *minute*."

Lucas flopped onto the sofa, leaned his head back, and shut his eyes.

Avery's tiny footsteps drew Rebecca's attention. She turned to her daughter and put up a hand to stop her, but Avery kept coming.

"Baby." Avery moved right beside them and tugged at the blanket. It fell away from the child's face, and Avery scowled. "Icky."

"Oh, dear Lord." Rebecca clutched her chest.

The half-naked little boy cried and clung onto her. His small body was covered in open, weeping pox.

Rebecca gaped at the horrid sight. "Avery. Go to your room."

"No."

"I said, go to your room!" Rebecca pointed a stiff finger in that direction.

Her daughter stuck out her lower lip, her chin vibrated, and the tears came. She ran down the hall and back to her bedroom. Exactly where Rebecca wished she'd stayed.

Rebecca took the boy to the kitchen and heated some water. She found some old diapers as well as clothes of Avery's that would fit him—though no boy would appreciate. But it didn't matter. He needed to be covered.

She placed a cool cloth on his forehead. "You poor child. You've got such a fever."

His chin quivered just like Avery's. He was a handsome boy, even with his blistered face. She'd never seen the pox up close like this, but to her understanding, small children overcame them quite well.

"Unlike adults," she mumbled. The reality of her situation stung. She feared for Avery, but the risk she'd taken herself by tending him was much greater.

She cleaned the boy and carefully dabbed at the many open sores, then dressed him. She wrapped him in a clean blanket and put him in the center of her bed.

He fussed and whimpered. She couldn't begin to imagine how uncomfortable he must be. It was unlikely he was hungry—not with such a fever—but he was most definitely tired. She spoke softly to him and calmed away his tears. It wasn't long before he fell asleep.

Avery had also stopped crying, but hadn't come out of her room. Rebecca glanced in to check on her and found her sitting on the floor with Moo Cow.

The child pointed a finger in the plush face. "Go room."

The sight tugged at Rebecca's insides. She needed to apologize to Avery for yelling, but she had something more pressing to do.

She marched to the living room and sat down hard in the chair beside the sofa.

Lucas hugged himself and shivered. "You got anymore blankets?"

"You're sick, too, aren't you?"

"Don't reckon so." His eyes slightly opened. "I'm just tired. I've been ridin' hard for three days. Can you get me a blanket?"

She went to the extra bedroom, yanked a quilt from the bed, and returned to Lucas. Part of her wanted to tell him to leave, but she'd never been cruel. She carefully lay the quilt atop him and he cuddled it up to his chin.

"Where's Caleb?" Lucas sneered. "It's him I wanna see."

"He's in the barn. One of our cows is birthin'."

Lucas grunted. "Figgers." He opened his eyes a bit wider. "You're lookin' might fine. Seems things is goin' good for ya."

Rebecca firmly folded her arms over her chest. "Why do you need my husband?"

The boy smirked—an image she'd not forgotten. "I brung him a present."

"What do you mean?"

"That nice little package I was carryin'. It's Caleb's."

"What?" Her heart seemed to stop beating. "You brought the child for Caleb?"

"It's *his*. Don't you understand?" Lucas's smirk turned into leering hate. "That boy is Caleb's bastard."

She grasped the arm of the chair. "You're lyin'. Caleb would've told me if—"

Lucas let out an awful-sounding cackle. "What? If he'd poked a woman before you?" He tried to lean toward her, but huffed a breath and dropped back against the cushions. "You don't know your husband. He ain't the man you thought."

Numbness started at Rebecca's head and worked its way to her feet. She couldn't move—couldn't *think*. She simply stared at Lucas.

A loud bawl brought her to her senses. She rapidly shook her head and stood. "The child needs me." She walked in a daze to her bedroom and peered down at the innocent boy lying on her bed.

Caleb's features stared back at her.

She stuck her head into the hallway. "What's his name?" she yelled to Lucas.

Lucas laughed. "Noah!"

Though disgusted that he took such pleasure in making her miserable, Rebecca disregarded him and focused on the child.

Noah.

Caleb had called out that very name one night. He'd said he'd had a dream. The incident had happened soon after the Larsen boy's first visit when Caleb had gone into town to question him. Lucas must have told Caleb about the child.

She eased onto the bed and picked him up. The sweet boy held onto her, but she could tell he was weak. It had been some time since he'd been properly cared for.

"Noah?" she whispered.

He blinked a few times and grinned. Incredible that a smile could come to the boy when he was so sick. His expression looked just like Caleb's.

"You have your pa's dark hair, too." Rebecca had fought off crying, but the reality hit so hard, she couldn't help it, and the tears came. "Lily must be your ma. It has to be her."

"Sissy." Noah patted her face.

Why would he say that?

She tried to lay him down again, but he clung on tight. His open sores brushed against her bare arms. She breathed the air he exhaled. Only a miracle would keep her from getting sick.

"Ma?" Avery crept across the floor and climbed onto the bed. "I bad?"

Rebecca was tempted to shoo her away again, but her daughter's sad face prevented her from doing it. "No. You did nothin' wrong," she whispered. "I'm sorry I yelled." She rocked Noah back and forth. "But this baby is sick, an' I don't want you to get sick, too. Understand?"

Her tiny brows moved up and down. "Get Pa."

Rebecca's world was crumbling around her, and her innocent daughter couldn't see it. Yet maybe that was for the best. Although Rebecca had lost faith in Caleb, Avery needed to believe in him.

Even so, Rebecca wanted to hear her husband's explanation about Noah.

The truth was bound to be painful, but knowing he'd lied hurt even worse.

Chapter 23

Caleb wiped his hands on an old rag, then stood back and watched.

This little calf wasn't the cow's first, so things had progressed well and without complication. No matter how many times Caleb witnessed a birthing, he appreciated the miracle.

Thoroughly licked clean, the calf rose up on shaky legs and easily found its mother's udder. Another sight to marvel at. The animal's natural instincts couldn't be denied.

"Avery's gonna love you." He grinned at the suckling calf, then headed to the house.

He was so eager to show his daughter the new life in the barn that he accidentally slammed the back door.

"Pa!"

Avery's excited voice added fuel to his happiness.

"No, Avery!" Rebecca yelled. "Stay here."

Rebecca never raised her voice to Avery. Something wasn't right.

Caleb followed the sounds of their voices and found them in his and Rebecca's bedroom. "What's wro—?" He snapped his mouth shut. "Where'd that baby come from?"

Avery grinned and pointed. "Noah."

"Noah?" Caleb couldn't breathe. "What . . .?" His mind raced in a hundred different directions. "How . . .?"

Rebecca cradled the toddler against her. "You best sit down, Caleb. You're awfully pale." She faced him, expressionless. "Lucas Larsen is in the livin' room. He brought the boy."

With his mind spinning, Caleb had to sit. He eased onto the edge of the bed. How much did Rebecca know?

Avery crawled into his lap. "Baby sick."

"Sick?"

Rebecca pulled the blanket away from the boy's face. "It's pox. I believe he's had it for some time. Lucas claims *he's* not sick, but my understandin' is that it can take a couple weeks before the blisters come out. Lucas looks wretched, but I have no sympathy for him."

"But why are you holdin' that child?"

She lifted her chin high. "Lucas nearly dropped him on the floor. He said he brought this boy to you. As a present." She turned to Avery. "Sweetheart, will you go to your room an' get Moo Cow for me?"

She happily obliged her ma and left the room.

Rebecca leaned close to Caleb. "Lucas said Noah is your child. Your *bastard*, as he put it."

"Becca, I—"

"Here." Avery climbed atop the bed and handed over her toy.

"Thank you." Rebecca patted the top of the stuffed cow's head. "Does the new calf look anythin' like Moo Cow?" She widened her eyes and forced a smile.

His dear wife was putting on a front for Avery's sake. "A bit." He swallowed the bile that had worked its way into his throat. "But we'll hafta wait till another day to see it. We all best stay inside for now."

Rebecca swayed with Noah. "Caleb? Have you ever had the pox?"

"Long time ago."

Her jaw tightened. "I haven't. An' as you know, Avery hasn't either."

"You didn't get 'em when we was little?"

"No." She sadly shook her head, and it broke his heart. "My folks kept me from such things. They thought they were doin' right by me, but I reckon they weren't."

He extended his arms. "I'll hold the baby. You shouldn't be so close to him."

"It's too late for that. I assume I'm already exposed."

"Don't say that." He took Noah from her. "There's a chance, you haven't gotten infected. I want you an' Avery to go to her room. Keep away from Noah *and* Lucas."

"Maybe we should go to the hotel."

"No." His head throbbed. How could this be happening? "If you *are* infected, we can't take the risk a passin' it on."

Heat from Noah's body penetrated the blanket. Caleb stared at the bundle in his arms.

Rebecca rose and took Avery by the hand. "We have plenty a time to talk 'bout all this later."

Guilt had never weighed so heavy. Caleb shut his eyes and shook his head.

"Caleb?" Rebecca set a hand on his arm. "Take care a that boy. All right?"

"I will."

Her sad eyes roamed over Noah's small frame, then she led Avery from the room.

Now alone with his son, Caleb tried to digest the situation.

The boy whimpered and scratched at his arms.

"No, son," Caleb whispered. "That won't help."

The boy looked up into his face. "Sissy?" He sniffled and pointed out the door.

"You mean Avery?" Caleb's heart beat hard. "You think she's your sister?"

"Sissy." He stuck out his lower lip and pointed again.

Caleb cupped a hand to his head. "We gotta get your fever down." He carried Noah into the kitchen and poured cool water into a large pan. Honestly, he needed the bathing tub, but didn't care to go to the barn to fetch it.

He stripped Noah bare, then set the pan on the floor. "It's kinda cold, but it'll help." He sat the child in it.

Noah's eyes popped wide and his face scrunched together, but he didn't cry. "Cold." He stared at Caleb for a moment, then slapped at the water. Caleb carefully scooped it with a cup and drizzled it all over his son's body.

It seemed as if the water not only helped with the fever, but Noah stopped trying to scratch at the sores. They were everywhere. Even inside his mouth. When Noah started to shiver, Caleb dried him off and put him in a clean diaper.

"I don't know if you've been taught to go 'thout these, but I don't wanna take a chance with you bein' sick an' all." He quickly calculated in his head and figured the boy to be about sixteen months.

"I cold." Noah reached for him.

Caleb didn't waste one second. He covered him with another dry towel and drew him close. "I can't believe you're here. You gotta get better." The boy wrapped his arms and legs around him as if horribly frightened.

Caleb tenderly patted his back. "*Please*, get better."

With Noah in his arms, Caleb headed for the living room.

Lucas had some explaining to do.

Caleb sat with Noah still clinging to him.

Lucas opened one eye. "Caleb?" He moaned and shifted on the sofa, then pushed himself partially upright. "I see the two a you met."

The instant he spoke, Noah's eyes widened. He shifted his body far away from Lucas and trembled.

Caleb leered at Lucas. "What did you do to my boy?"

"Already actin' like his pa, huh?" He grunted out a laugh.

"You're insane." Caleb turned his body enough to shield his son from Lucas. "Did you drag Noah all the way from the cove?"

"I wouldn't call it draggin'. But it wasn't a fun ride. The little brat squalled the whole time." Lucas curled his lip and scowled. "I told you someday I'd bring him to show your pretty wife."

"Damn you. He's sick. He should've been left where he was bein' cared for. You coulda killed him."

Lucas shrugged. "I don't care. Cuz a him, my ma's dyin'. It'll serve him right if he dies, too."

"He's a *baby*. Don't you have a heart?"

Lucas scooted down fully flat on the sofa. "Reckon I do. It's poundin' in my chest right now. I feel awful. Haven't slept decent in days."

"Poor you." Caleb didn't even try to hide his disgust. "Does Lily know 'bout Noah an' your ma bein' sick?"

Lucas sneered. "Lily's still all you care 'bout, ain't she?"

"Does she know?" Caleb persisted.

"Course she does. She got a telegram just like me. But she had a long way to travel. All the way from Asheville."

"Asheville?" *She's so close.*

"Yep. I passed her an' her driver comin' here." Lucas snickered. "But I made sure they didn't see us. It wasn't easy keepin' Noah quiet. But it woulda spoiled everythin' if she'd a found us."

"How can you be so cruel?"

"Don't talk to me 'bout bein' cruel. You've been horrid to that poor wife a yours, lyin' 'bout everythin'. I did her a favor by bringin' Noah here. But don't worry. Once Lily gets home an' sees Noah ain't there, she'll know where to come lookin' for him.

Then we'll all have a nice, big party. We can all can get to know each other."

Caleb was tempted to pummel him, but squeezed his eyes shut and forced himself to calm down.

"Truth really hurts when it comes to Lily, don't it?" Lucas's words took another jab.

Noah's head popped up. "Sissy?"

Lucas snorted out a laugh.

Caleb looked from him to Noah, then back at Lucas again. "Why does he keep sayin' *sissy*?"

"Cuz I was talkin' 'bout Lily. He thinks she's his sister. Isaac an' Horace talk 'bout her a lot. They cry all the time cuz they think our ma's mean. They'd rather have Lily. My family is a mess cuz you came in an' ruined it." He readjusted his blankets. "I'm tired. I wanna sleep."

"Fine. Go on an' sleep. It'll be easier to turn you over to the law."

Lucas's head lifted. "What's that s'posed to mean?"

"Now that my wife knows my secret, you have nothin' to hang over my head to keep me from tellin' what you done to Ableman. You should be locked up." Caleb rubbed Noah's small back. "I used to wanna protect you, cuz you kept Ableman from gettin' his hands on Lily. But you endangered our son. I won't let you hurt anyone else in my family."

Lucas waved a single hand and let his head fall against the cushions. "I don't care no more. Do what you hafta." He shut his eyes, then yanked the blanket up to his chin.

"Caleb?" Rebecca's soft whisper carried through the room.

Caleb turned to find her standing in the hallway. He got up, hoisted Noah onto his shoulder, and moved within several feet of Rebecca. "Are you okay?"

"No." She'd never looked sadder. "I heard what you told Lucas. All this time you didn't tell the law 'bout him because you were afraid I'd find out the truth. You didn't want me to know 'bout you an' Lily."

He stared at her, dumfounded. "I . . . I didn't know how to tell you. Lily an' me . . . that is . . . I didn't know 'bout Noah. She never told me. An' when Lucas did, I didn't fully believe him."

"You lied to me straight out when I asked if you'd ever had a woman. An' the thing is, I wouldn't a cared if you'd said yes, not when you were marryin' *me*." She shook her head and furrowed her brow. "I'm scared there are other things you've kept from me. I feel like I don't know you at all." She leaned against the wall and rested her head there. Her features had become vacant. "Does your ma know 'bout Noah?"

As hard as it was to tell the truth, Caleb was done lying. "I told her what Lucas said, so yes, she knows. But she assumed he was lyin'."

"That means she also knows 'bout you an' Lily."

He nodded, but couldn't utter a word.

Rebecca stared blankly forward. "I trusted her—even more so than you. I knew it was wrong to doubt you all the time, but I finally understand why that voice inside me told me things weren't right. I started thinkin' I was crazy. *Foolish*. But now, knowin' I've been lied to over an' over again . . ." She breathed in and stood tall. "I'll stay with Avery in her room till we know whether or not we'll get the pox. If I somehow avoided bein' infected, I'll take Avery with me an' move into the hotel."

"No, Becca. Please don't say that. You two are my life."

"No, we're not. Your life was lived with someone else, an' you hold the proof in your arms. I'm done tryin' to be your wife. I understand now. You've always wanted someone else." She walked into Avery's room and shut the door.

Caleb hugged Noah to his aching chest. He never meant to hurt Rebecca this way. But what hurt the most was that she'd spoken the truth.

He'd always wanted Lily.

Even so, it would tear him apart if Rebecca left with Avery. He'd fallen in love with the child from the moment she'd come into the world. He was the only pa she knew. It wouldn't just break *his* heart to have her taken from him, it would break *hers* as well.

He trudged to his room and lay down on the bed with his son.

The boy curled his small body against him and nestled his head over Caleb's heart.

Though still feverish, at least his breathing was steady. Caleb heard no sign of rattling in Noah's chest. Even covered in ugly blisters, his son was perfect. The result of Lily's and his love. Nothing could be more beautiful.

"I never wanna let you go," he whispered and kissed the top of Noah's head.

Caleb lay back on the pillow and shut his eyes. The house had become completely quiet.

The stress of the situation had worn on Caleb emotionally and physically. He tried to think everything through, but no solution he could come up with had a happy ending.

Chapter 24

Rebecca gently moved Avery's small arms and inched away from her. It had taken a while to get her to nap again, but Rebecca had sung to her to reassure her all was well.

Nothing was further from the truth.

Truth.

It didn't exist in their home.

She carefully opened the bedroom door and crept out.

If only she hadn't been so needy when Caleb had arrived in Waynesville. Had she been a stronger person, she might have seen through his façade.

She glanced into the living room. Lucas lay sprawled out on the sofa with his mouth hanging wide open. He snored something fierce.

She turned and headed the short distance down the hallway to Caleb's and her bedroom. One she would never occupy again.

The sight before her pierced her heart in an unusual way. Father and son lying side by side. Lily had given Caleb the son he deserved. The child Rebecca had been unable to bear.

The two looked so content. So peaceful.

Rebecca was rightfully angry with Caleb, yet she still loved him. He'd been a part of her life forever, and she couldn't turn her back on him now. Even so, she couldn't continue playing the role of his wife any longer. She'd have been smarter to remain his sister.

She tiptoed to the kitchen and poured a glass of water. A loaf of bread on the counter caught her eye, but she couldn't bring herself to eat a bite.

It was suppertime and although she wasn't hungry, she needed to feed Avery.

Caleb, too.

She pulled out a chair from the table and sat. Sighing, she put her elbows on the tabletop and leaned her head on one hand. She certainly didn't feel like cooking.

"Becca?" Caleb walked in and took the seat across from her. "I thought you was nappin'."

"I couldn't. Seemed silly to sleep midday." She kept her eyes focused on the table and off him. "I sang to Avery till she fell asleep. I think she's confused. She doesn't understand all that's happened."

"She ain't the only one." He reached across the table and tried to take her hand, but she pulled away.

"Don't. Please?" She looked him straight in the eye to drive her point.

He drew his hand to himself. "I hate seein' you like this. I know it's my fault." He turned away. "I'm *always* to blame."

"Stop feelin' sorry for yourself. Your biggest fault is that you've never grown up an' accepted responsibility." She leaned toward him and lowered her voice. "You put a child in a woman an' left her to fend for herself. If you loved her so much, why would you do such a thing? No decent *man* would."

His fists tightened. "It's long an' complicated. But I swear I did what I thought was best."

"How could it be?" She leaned back and folded her arms. "Go on an' tell me this long, complicated story. I want to hear it."

"Becca . . ." He pinched his lips together and shook his head. "I can't tell it. Not now."

She scooted her chair back and stood. "Fine. An' I can't cook right now. I'm goin' out to swing for a spell."

Needing to distance herself from him, she marched from the house. If she hadn't left right then and there, she very well could've slapped him.

* * *

Being told he hadn't grown up and accepted responsibility didn't set well with Caleb. But the only way to make Rebecca understand his actions would be by telling her what he'd done to Abraham. Once she knew that, she might accept his explanations, but how could they ever reconcile?

To complicate matters more, if what Lucas said was true, Lily would arrive any day.

Caleb's insides tumbled. Though hungry, it was more than that. A lot more. He couldn't imagine having both Lily and Rebecca together in the same house. He wouldn't know how to act. And if Lily despised him as much as Rebecca did at the moment, he didn't have a prayer.

So, what would a responsible adult do in this situation?

He internally chided Rebecca for saying what she had. Hadn't he proved his manhood? Couldn't Rebecca see how hard he worked the farm? The place had been nonproducing before he'd taken it over. Now it thrived. They had abundant crops and plenty of livestock.

The new calf . . .

He'd promised to show Avery the newborn. It couldn't hurt to take her outside to see it. As Rebecca had said, it could be weeks before they knew if they were infected. As long as they stayed close to home and didn't come into contact with others, they'd do no harm. Besides, he couldn't expect to keep his daughter cooped up in her room for that length of time.

He'd likely need to cook supper himself, but it would have to wait.

He got to his feet and went after his daughter. As he neared her room, he heard her softly singing to her stuffed cow.

He opened the door enough to see her.

"Moo, moo, moo. Cow go moo, moo, moo." Her sweet repetitive tune warmed Caleb's heart. Something he needed.

"Avery?" he whispered and pushed the door wide. "Wanna go see the baby cow?"

She tossed her toy on the floor, ran to Caleb, and lifted her arms. Her actions said more than any words.

Before going out, Caleb peeked in on Noah to make certain he was still asleep. He hadn't budged from the spot Caleb had left him.

"We can't stay out long," Caleb whispered. "We gotta keep our eyes on Noah. But I want you to see the calf."

"Baby cow."

"That's right." He kissed her cheek and carried her outside to the barn.

The calf no longer shook on his lean legs. He stood strong and steady. Caleb pointed. "Ain't he fine?"

Avery grinned. "I pet cow?"

"All right. But you gotta be gentle."

He took her close to the calf. Its mother came near and nudged Caleb's leg. He stroked her head to ease her. "Don't fret. We won't hurt your baby."

Avery copied his action and pet the cow, then reached for the calf. She brushed her fingers along its nose.

The mother cow let out a moo.

Caleb chuckled. "Its ma don't like us touchin' her baby. Mas are protective of their young. They won't let 'em outta their sight."

Avery cuddled onto his shoulder, then pointed toward the house. "Baby."

"You're right. We best get back an' check on Noah."

Avery waved goodbye to the cows and they headed back toward the house.

If she'd been a little older, she probably would've asked about Noah's ma, and why she wasn't with him.

No matter what happened when Lily arrived, Caleb would do all he could to keep from confusing Avery more than she already was.

The only comfort he had was in knowing that children as young as Avery and Noah wouldn't remember these days. Adults didn't have that benefit. Too many painful things remained in Caleb's mind.

"Ma!" Avery called out. "Swing."

Avery wiggled and twisted until he set her down. She ran toward her ma on the swing.

Rebecca slowed to a stop. "Come on." She patted her lap and Avery climbed up.

Before getting it going again, Rebecca faced Caleb.

Their eyes locked and heaviness tugged at his heart. No matter how many times he told her he was sorry, he could never make things right again. But somehow, they had to find a way to work through this.

A sad smile lifted Rebecca's lips. She pushed with her feet and got the swing moving. Avery held on tight. Her giggles filled the air.

This was one memory Caleb wanted to hold onto forever. The two looked so beautiful and happy. He didn't want to consider the idea that they'd come down with the pox, yet the possibility hung over them. Dark and dismal. Nothing like the clear blue sky above them now.

He glanced their way a final time and returned inside.

* * *

Eggs, bacon, and biscuits might not be the best supper, but Caleb threw it together to make a meal.

Rebecca had come in with Avery soon after he'd started cooking. After washing Avery's hands and face, she took the child into her room and hadn't come out since.

These next few weeks were bound to be painful.

Lucas trudged into the kitchen. "You can cook?"

Caleb kept his eyes on the bacon. "I get by." He wished he could feel something more than disgust for Lily's brother. After all, they'd been friends at one time.

Lucas stretched and rubbed the back of his neck. "That sofa don't sleep too good."

"If you'd like, you can sleep in our guestroom." Caleb would probably regret saying it, but he felt the need to try and make things better between them. "I reckon you ain't got nowhere else to go. Am I right?"

He jerked out a chair and sat down. "I thought I was goin' to the county jail. What happened to gettin' the law?"

"I was angry." He turned the bacon over with a fork. "Still am, but I've calmed down some. Noah's sleepin' well an' seems to be gettin' better. Till I know for sure what's gonna happen with you an' my girls, I ain't goin' nowhere."

Lucas thrummed his fingers on the tabletop. "I'm fine. Like I said before, I'm just tired. I ain't gonna get the pox."

"You've had them before?"

"No. But that don't mean nothin'. If I was sick, I'd know it."

Caleb gave him a quick glance. The boy was as cocky as ever —self-assured and angry. "Are you hungry?"

"Some. I s'pose I can eat a bite or two." He tapped his feet on the floor and kept drumming the table with his fingers.

"You nervous 'bout sumthin'? You keep fidgetin'." Caleb put the bacon on a plate, then cracked some eggs into the hot grease.

"I ain't nervous. Just restless." He smacked the table hard, then crossed his arms. "My ma's probably dead by now."

Caleb flipped the eggs. Now he knew what was truly troubling Lucas. As hard a front as the boy put on, at one time he'd shown a lot of love for his family. "Are you sure she was that sick? Ill enough to die?"

"Yep. Pa said she got lung fever. It started with them pox, then kept on from there."

"You said Noah gave it to her. How'd that happen?"

Caleb set the eggs on two separate plates, then put a few slices of bacon beside them. He placed one plate in front of Lucas, then set the other one down for himself. He'd already put biscuits in a basket at the center of the table.

He handed Lucas a fork. "There's strawberry preserves in that jar. My ma an' Becca made 'em."

Lucas shoveled the eggs into his mouth, then stuffed an entire piece of bacon in along with them.

Caleb took his time eating. "I thought you said you wasn't very hungry."

"I lied. I ain't eaten in three days." He nabbed a biscuit and smeared on a glob of jam. "You said you wanna know how Noah got the pox?"

Caleb nodded and chewed on some bacon.

"Ma didn't like tendin' him. He gave her all sorts a trouble. So, she took him to a woman what has two other kids. They was sick, but my folks didn't know it. Noah came home from there an' passed it on. Isaac an' Horace is sick, too. But I reckon they'll live."

It seemed strange that Mrs. Larsen would have someone else watch Noah. None of it made much sense. "What 'bout your pa an' Violet?"

"Pa had pox when he was young. So'd Lily." When he said her name, his lip curled. "That's right, when she shows up you won't hafta worry 'bout her gettin' sick." He stuffed another large bite of biscuit into his mouth. "That should make you happy," he said through a mouthful of food.

"An' Violet? Is she all right?"

"Right as rain. She got married. An' surprise, surprise, she's already gonna have a baby." He grunted. "Pa went an' warned her to stay away."

"That's good. So, she still lives in the cove?"

"Yep. Married her a one-legged farmer. Slim pickin's 'round there." His eyes narrowed. "Neither a my sisters ever had any sense in choosin' a decent man."

Caleb set his fork down. "Why do you do that?"

"What?"

"I'm tryin' all I can to be nice to you, but you ain't makin' it easy."

Lucas stuck his nose in the air. "Why should I?"

"Because I'm givin' you a second chance. What you done hurt my wife. But I can't put all the blame on you. I shoulda set things right a long time ago." He leaned across the table. "I know I hurt you, an' I also know you're achin' inside over losin' your ma. But you wanna put on this tough front to prove you're some kind a big man. I remember the boy I taught how to hunt, an' how to make arrows an' scout for deer. What happened to change you?"

"I grew up." He sat back in his chair and stared at Caleb. "Do you know what it's like to have a pa who'd rather be with his daughter than his son?"

"No."

"I was the oldest boy. Pa shoulda been teachin' me how to take over the farm. But he taught Lily. Praised her all the time for what she done. I was always an afterthought. Then you come along an' you was good to me. Did all them things you said. But Lily took you away, too. You forgot me just like my pa."

Finally, it all made sense. "I know you love your pa. If not, you wouldn't a saved him when he got sick on that moonshine. You were the one who brought him in the house."

Lucas smirked. "An' you gave him the medicine that made him throw up. *You* saved him, not me." He hissed air out his nose. "Didn't you ever wonder how his moonshine got tainted?"

"I assumed sumthin' bad got in it."

"Mysteriously got in there, huh?" Lucas grunted and shook his head. "You ain't too smart. Since we're bein' all honest here, I put lye in that bottle. I *wanted* him to drink it."

Caleb had thought he was making progress with Lucas, but this revelation sent everything spiraling downward. It seemed there were no limits to the boy's callous acts. "You know how poisonous lye is, don't you?"

"That's why I put it in there. I knew he'd drink up all that moonshine, an' I wanted him dead. An' you know why? Cuz I thought maybe then you'd stay an' take his place. You was strong, an' Pa was weak."

"You're heartless."

Lucas gave his plate a shove. "No, I'm tired. Reckon I'll go get in that bed you offered." He stood and walked away.

Caleb pondered every single word that had come from the boy. He waited a short while, and once he knew Lucas was settled in the guestroom, Caleb crept to the door and locked it from the outside. He wasn't about to risk any further harm to his family.

Chapter 25

Between sleeping on the hard ground for three nights and being jostled by Stardust for three full days, every bone in Gideon's body ached.

All that kept him going were thoughts of Violet, their coming baby, and poor little Noah.

He'd hoped that he might happen on Lucas and the baby along the way, but he didn't have such luck.

Now in Waynesville, he prayed that they'd been right about where Lucas would take the child. But he somehow had to locate Caleb Henry. If Noah wasn't there, Gideon would have to return to Violet empty-handed. Something he didn't want to do. It would break her heart and his along with it.

He rode slowly down the main street of town.

Stardust tossed her head.

"It's all right, girl." Gideon patted her side. "I see a water trough." He led her to the front of a hotel where the trough was.

Aside from his travels during the war, he'd never been to many towns outside of Tennessee. But most every hotel accommodated both men and animals.

He'd kept his crutch tied in a fancy strap Violet had come up with. She had more smarts than him for such things.

He loosened the strap, grabbed the crutch, and carefully dismounted.

"Ugh." Simply standing hurt.

What he wouldn't give for a long soak in a hot tub of water.

After letting Stardust drink her fill, he guided her to a post and tethered her. Maybe someone in the hotel would know where to find Caleb.

He glanced down at his dirty clothes. Surely, he smelled wretched. But hopefully, folks here would be kind and disregard his appearance, as well as his odor. In this particular case, missing a leg could come in handy. Folks tended to sympathize with injured men.

He made his way to the front desk.

A woman sat behind it with a book in hand. She lifted her head, when Gideon cleared his throat.

"Yes? Need a room?"

"No'm." Gideon smiled as politely as he could. "It's important I find someone what lives here."

She sat taller and peered over the desk. For a brief second, her eyes rested on where his absent leg should've been, then she looked up and met his gaze with an expression of sympathy he'd seen many times before. "Lose it in the war?"

"Yes'm."

"Terrible, wasn't it?"

"That it was." Again, he cleared his throat. "Ma'am do you know where I might find Caleb Henry?"

She cocked her head to one side. "You a friend?"

"Well . . . I ain't never met him, but my wife knows him well. It's important that I see him right away."

"Hmm." She eyed him up and down. "Tell you what. I'll fetch his ma. If she feels your reasons are fittin', she can tell you where he is."

"His ma?"

"That's right. She lives here, an' she's a fine woman. So you best have come for honorable purposes." The woman set her book aside and stood. "I'll be back quicker than you can shake a leg. That is—well . . ." Red-faced, she scurried away.

Gideon hadn't taken offense. Her embarrassment actually eased him a mite.

He moved to a long bench, sat, and waited.

The desk clerk soon returned with another woman, presumably Caleb's ma. Though she had gray hair, she by no means looked old. She kept her long hair braided down one side and it fell across her front, almost to her waist. Comely for her age, that was for sure.

Gideon pushed himself up from the bench and nodded. "Hello, ma'am."

She studied him, then smiled. "Mrs. Iverson told me you're lookin' for my son, Caleb. What's your business with him?"

Gideon gulped. Mrs. Iverson hovered close and didn't appear to be going anywhere. "Ma'am, my business is of a personal nature. Can we speak in private?"

Mrs. Henry motioned for Mrs. Iverson to leave them. Once the desk clerk skittered away, Caleb's ma gestured to the door. "Why don't we go outside an' talk?"

"Fine idea." Gideon hobbled in that direction.

He hadn't prepared himself for *this*. What would he tell her?

I've come searchin' for a baby your son sired what was kidnapped by his mean uncle?

No. That wouldn't fly.

Gideon would have to just start at the beginning and pray she showed some sort of understanding.

"So . . ." Mrs. Henry stopped and faced him on the pathway. "How do you know Caleb? Did you serve with him in the war?"

"No'm. I ain't never met him. My wife knows him."

"Oh?" She jutted her chin. "Who's your wife?"

"Her name's Violet. Maiden name was Larsen."

Mrs. Henry's eyes grew wider than a full moon. "Larsen? Any kin to . . . *Lily*?" She whispered the name.

Thank goodness she knows who I'm talkin' 'bout.

He blew out a relieved breath. "Lily's her sister."

"I see. But why do you need to find Caleb?" Mrs. Henry fanned her face with one hand.

"It's a mite sensitive, but—ah, heck. I'll just spit it out. A bad case a the chickenpox has come to the cove. That's where I'm from—Cades Cove. My wife's family got it real bad. Truth be told, her ma's dyin'."

Mrs. Henry clutched her chest. "Go on . . ."

"Well, one a her boys—that is—our *nephew* was taken by Lucas. My brother-in-law."

She held up a hand. "You said Lucas. Lucas Larsen?"

"You know him?"

"Yes. Much as I hate to say it. He's a wretched creature." Her brows drew together. "You said he took your nephew? Who's child is he?"

"Um . . ." Gideon's skin felt as if it had been lit on fire. "I . . . um."

"Never mind." She shut her eyes and frowned. "The boy's Lily's son. Ain't that right?"

"Yes'm. But how—?"

"I know many things. Lucas told Caleb the child existed, but I didn't believe it."

"Oh, he exists all right. But he's sick as can be. The only place we all figgered Lucas would take him is to Caleb. His . . ." Gideon snapped his lips shut.

"His pa," Mrs. Henry calmly said.

Gideon nodded.

Her eyes opened large again, but in a different way. As if she'd come to realize something.

"Oh, my," she muttered. "If the baby has the pox . . ." She grabbed Gideon's arm. "We've gotta go there at once. My grandchild will be exposed. Her ma, too."

Gideon pointed behind him. "My horse is over yonder. How far is it to their place?"

"Not far. I usually walk, but we don't have time. I'll borrow Mr. Iverson's buggy. You can follow me." She sped off before Gideon could reply. He didn't know women her age could move so fast.

He hurried back to Stardust and mounted.

Things had gone better than he'd expected, but until they found Noah, his heart wouldn't rest.

* * *

"Unlock this right now!" Lucas beat on the bedroom door.

Caleb had expected him to wake up a lot sooner than he had. He'd slept through the night and half of the morning. "Stop your fussin'." Caleb inserted the key and turned it.

Lucas yanked the door wide. "You had no right lockin' me in here."

"I had every right. You confessed to poisonin' your own pa. I'm takin' a risk havin' you in my home. So, when I sleep, you'll be locked in here. Either that, or I'll boot you out on your own."

Lucas squirmed. "I gotta use the outhouse."

"Fine. Go. But I'll be watchin' you."

The boy sprinted off.

"Pa!"

Caleb froze. The cry hadn't come from Avery. She and Rebecca were outside. It could only be one other soul.

Caleb rushed to his bedroom. Noah sat up in the center of the bed with his arms stretched toward him. "Pa hold?"

Maybe the child referred to every man as pa. Just like most women were sissy.

No matter, Caleb lifted him from the bed and held him. "Your fever's not so high today." He stroked the boy's head. "That's good."

"Eat?"

"You're hungry? That's even better."

Caleb carried him to the kitchen. His pock-covered face still looked a sight, but his behavior indicated he was on the mend. Especially if his appetite had returned.

"Can you sit in a highchair?"

Silly question. The boy was plenty big enough.

Caleb scooted Avery's highchair close to the table and set Noah in it.

Eggs seemed like a good idea. They'd go easy on the boy's stomach. So Caleb scrambled two eggs with a bit of milk and poured them into a frying pan. They didn't take long to cook.

Noah watched every move he made.

When Caleb set the food on a plate in front of Noah, he grinned.

Caleb blew on the eggs to cool them and the child giggled. Another wonderful sign of healing.

"Go on. You can use your fingers. An' if you're anythin' like Avery, you'll wear some a them eggs in your hair."

Noah reached for the eggs, but jumped when Lucas came back inside and slammed the door. He hovered over Noah.

Noah cowered and reached for Caleb. The poor boy's chin quivered.

Caleb jerked his head toward the living room. "Go on, Lucas. My boy don't like bein' 'round you, an' he needs to eat."

"Fine." Lucas grunted. "I know when I ain't wanted."

He left, and Noah's demeanor brightened again.

Caleb pulled a chair up next to him. "He won't hurt you. I'll see to it." He cupped a hand over his son's head. "You can eat.

They're good." Caleb grabbed a small piece of egg and popped it into his own mouth. "Mmm. Yummy eggs."

"Mmm," Noah repeated, then grabbed a fistful. They squirted out from between his little fingers, but a great deal ended up in his mouth.

Caleb feared they might irritate the sores there, but Noah didn't fuss and kept on eating.

Raised voices came from outside. Caleb peered out the kitchen window and discovered his ma and a one-legged stranger talking to Rebecca and Avery.

Caleb wasn't about to leave Noah alone with Lucas, so he stayed where he was but kept watching the interchange.

His ma appeared to be crying. Rebecca pointed at the house and the man and his ma headed toward him.

Caleb returned to Noah's side. "I reckon your gramma knows 'bout you. All you gotta do is smile an' she'll love you forever."

Noah stuffed more eggs in his mouth.

The door squeaked open. Noah turned in his chair and grinned.

Caleb had no idea if the boy had understood a word he'd said, but Noah couldn't have displayed a finer expression.

His ma held a hand to her heart and knelt beside him "Oh, my goodness. Aside from all the blisters, he looks exactly like you when you was a baby." Tears trickled onto her cheeks. "Caleb, what are you gonna do?"

"Hey, Mrs. Henry." Lucas walked in smirking, then stumbled backward when he spotted the one-legged man. "Gideon?"

"Surprised to see me, Lucas?" Gideon glared at him, then crossed to Caleb's ma and placed a hand on Noah's head. "Violet's gonna be so relieved to know you're fine."

"Sissy!" Noah reached for Gideon.

"That's what he calls my wife." Gideon's cheeks reddened. "You must be Caleb. I'm Gideon Myers. Violet's husband."

"Good to meet you." Caleb gestured to a chair. "Please, sit. I know there's a lot to talk 'bout."

"Yes, there is," his ma said and took her own seat.

Lucas waved them away. "Count me out. I've seen an' heard all I care to."

"You should never a taken this boy," Gideon harshly said. "What were you thinkin'?"

"Don't know. But ain't we havin' fun?" Lucas strode off.

Gideon fisted his hand on top of the table. "Sometimes I'd like to whup that boy."

"Stand in line," Caleb muttered.

"Forget him," his ma said. "There are more important things to discuss." She placed two fingers under Noah's chin, lifted his head, and examined his lesions. "At least they're crustin' over. I can get some calamine lotion from Doc Garrison to stop the itchin'."

Caleb thought it was a fine idea, but . . . "You reckon it's okay for you to leave now that you've been exposed?"

"I've had the chickenpox an' I doubt my just bein' near this baby will have me passin' it on to others. Even so, I'll keep my distance from folks. But someone's gotta get medicine for this sweet boy."

Rebecca walked in holding Avery's hand. "Are we interruptin'?"

"Course not." His ma reached out to her. "This is your home. Where you belong." She emphasized her final words and looked from Rebecca to Caleb.

"That's right," he said. "How are you feelin'?"

"We're fine. I came in to fix sumthin' for Avery to eat." She eyed Noah. "Seems *he's* doin' better."

Noah leaned his head way back and reached for her. "Sissy."

Avery giggled, which prompted one from Noah.

Rebecca lifted Noah from the highchair. "I'll clean him up. He smells like he needs changin'."

"But . . ." Caleb held up a hand. "You shouldn't be close to him."

"It's too late for that now. 'Sides, I can't expect you to do everythin' 'round here." She left, with the boy nestled against her.

Avery climbed into Caleb's lap, then pointed at the stove. "Eggs?"

"I'll fix you some." He passed her off to his ma.

"My," she mumbled. "This is quite a mess."

The room fell silent.

Chapter 26

Gideon had always thought Violet's family had tense moments, but the tension in Caleb's house went beyond anything he'd experienced. Everyone acted as nice as can be—with the exception of Lucas—but Gideon could tell there was much left unsaid.

He couldn't return Noah to the cove while he was sick. Not to mention, he'd not exactly figured out how he'd get him there. It had been hard enough staying atop Stardust alone, he couldn't manage with a child in his arms. He and Violet hadn't really thought the whole plan through. Worse yet, how was he going to be around her again after being exposed to the pox? It definitely put a damper in his plans.

Since Lily was on her way, she'd see to Noah. And that in itself would add more fuel to the flaming Henry fire. The strain her presence would put on the family might snap it in half.

He'd gotten his wish for a hot bath. Thanks to Rebecca. She was kind and pleasant, but he could tell she'd had her heart broken. Such a shame for a decent woman like her.

As for sleep, he was given the sofa, which suited him fine. Far better than the hard ground.

Mrs. Henry fussed over Lucas having her room, but when Caleb explained that it was necessary to be able to lock him in at night, she quit complaining. She shared a bed with Rebecca and Avery.

They all survived one full day with each other, but now that Gideon knew Noah was being cared for, he wanted to get home to Violet. He missed her terribly.

He'd allow himself a good night's sleep, but he ached for home.

It felt like Gideon had just shut his eyes, when he opened them again to bright daylight. He'd slept like a rock. Didn't stir one bit and woke in the same position he'd fallen asleep in.

"Mornin'," Caleb said. "Feel like givin' me a hand with the livestock?"

Gideon sat up and stretched. "I'd like that. 'Sides, I need to check on Stardust. I appreciate you lettin' me put her in your barn for the night."

"I reckon she'll enjoy grazin' more. I got a new calf I'd like you to see. You raise cattle?"

"Nope. Only crops." Gideon grabbed his crutch and stood. "Used to wanna be a rancher, but . . ." He gestured downward. "That changed."

"You seem to manage *ridin'* just fine. Came a long way to fetch Noah. You're a good man, Gideon." Caleb headed toward the back door. "C'mon. My ma's gonna look after Noah. You an' me can work up an appetite an' have a big breakfast later. I ain't a bad cook." He grinned and walked out the door.

Gideon followed.

Violet had expressed extreme dislike for Caleb. Gideon understood why. After all, the man got Lily pregnant and left her. But from what he saw of Caleb, he was decent. Not only hardworking, he definitely loved the children.

There were always two sides to a story, and Gideon wanted to know Caleb's.

By the time Gideon got to the barn, Caleb was already hard at work cleaning up after the horses.

"I've shoveled more manure in my lifetime than I care to think 'bout," he said with a laugh.

"Try doin' that with only one leg." Gideon smiled and made his way to Stardust's stall. "It takes a while to get your balance."

Caleb's brows wove. He bent one leg and held it up off the ground, then tried scooping a shovelful. He teetered and nearly fell.

Gideon laughed. "See what I mean. Takes practice." He opened the mare's stall and guided her out to the field. "Go on an' run." He patted her rump and she wasted no time. Soon, her head was bent low in a field of grass.

He returned inside to Caleb. "My horse likes it here."

"Most do. Plenty a grass. Lots a water. Other horses to run 'round with." He grinned again, then sobered. "You must think I'm awful."

Gideon sat down on a bale of straw. "Why do you say that?"

Caleb huffed and leaned against his shovel. "You don't know me from Adam, but I feel comfortable with you. Like I've known you forever. Maybe because we both fell in love with a Larsen girl."

"I can't believe you're sayin' that so openly. You bein' married to Rebecca an' all."

"Like I said. You must think I'm awful. But you know 'bout me an' Lily, an' it's obvious we have a child together. I wanted you to know that I truly loved her. If I'd known 'bout Noah, I wouldn't a married Becca."

"So, why did you?"

"It's complicated. But she's a good woman an' I hate I hurt her." He tapped the shovel on the ground a few times. "You're lucky to be married to Violet. She's a special girl. Beautiful, too."

"Don't hafta tell me that." Gideon smiled just thinking of her. "Did you know she's gonna have a baby?"

"Yep. Lucas told me. Congratulations. You'll be a great pa." Caleb fidgeted with the shovel. "So, you wanna see that calf? I got him an' his ma penned up out back for the time bein'. Soon, they'll join the others in the open field."

"I'd like that."

"C'mon, then." Caleb headed toward the back of the barn. He pushed open a large door that led to a fenced-in area. Plenty big enough to give them room to roam.

Gideon leaned against the fence and smiled as the cow nuzzled the calf. "Incredible sight to see."

"Yep. I've known ranchers that describe the awful sound the cows make when they take the calves from 'em." Caleb gazed upward and his eyes misted over. "How did Lily ever part with Noah?"

Gideon had no doubt that Caleb still cared. "I didn't see it myself, but Violet told me it was awful. Lily stopped eatin' an' withdrew from everyone. It didn't get much better when they sent her to St. Louis. But you'll be glad to know that the family she's been with in Asheville has treated her decent."

Caleb sniffed and swiped a hand over his eyes. "That's good." He took a long breath. "Her family was kind to me. I loved each an' every one a them. Even Lucas." He kicked at the ground, then again wiped his eyes. "I hated to hear 'bout their ma. I worry for Isaac an' Horace."

"Violet an' me will help look after 'em. An' I'm sure Lily will, too. I hope you understand that once she gets her hands on Noah, she won't let him go again. I know he's your son an' all, but you won't be able to keep him."

Caleb put his back to Gideon and held onto the fence. "I'm aware. Reckon I aim to lose everythin'."

Gideon went up behind him and placed a firm hand on his shoulder. "Noah will always be your son. I know Lily. She won't shut you out a his life."

"My ma wants me to work things out with Becca. I know it's best. I married her an' made a commitment. Becca plans to move out, but I can't let her just throw it all away."

"Do you love her?"

"Becca?" Caleb turned and looked Gideon in the eye.

"Yes. Your *wife*."

"Course I do. She's been part a my life forever."

"What 'bout Lily? You still love her, too."

Caleb's eyes shifted downward. "Yep. I do." He puffed out a burst of air. "Not good, huh?"

"Nope. I'm glad I ain't in your shoes." He patted Caleb's back, then stood silently beside him.

He meant what he said wholeheartedly. Gideon was grateful he'd never loved more than one woman. He wouldn't wish that kind of complication on anyone. Violet alone had always filled his heart. Maybe if she saw Caleb through his eyes at this very moment, she might feel the pity for him that Gideon felt. And though Caleb hadn't told him everything that led to his marrying Rebecca, Gideon was certain Caleb had made his decision in an honorable way.

Caleb stared at the sky. "Will you do sumthin' for me, Gideon? I know it's askin' a lot, but I could sure use your help."

"What is it?"

Caleb turned around and leaned back on the fence. "Stay with us till Lily gets here. Things could get . . . *strange*."

Gideon scratched the back of his head. "It'll probably be a day or two 'fore she comes." He wanted to leave, but he'd come here to help. Yes, he'd been sent for Noah, but maybe by helping Caleb, it would help the child, too. "If I can get word to Violet that all is well, then I don't mind stayin'."

"Ma's goin' into town to get medicine from Doc Garrison. I'll ask her to send a telegram."

"Thank you." Gideon extended his hand.

Caleb firmly grabbed hold and shook it.

Gideon couldn't deny that he liked Caleb Henry. If only things had been different. Gideon missed his brothers, and Caleb would've been a fine brother-in-law.

* * *

Caleb had great respect for Gideon. Not only was he a fine man, he'd overcome the loss of a limb and seemed to be coping well with it.

Gideon walked over to the woodpile and picked up the axe. Caleb came close to stopping him, then watched in amazement as Gideon split a large log into smaller pieces. When he finished, he wiped his brow with the back of his hand.

"I reckon there ain't nothin' you can't do," Caleb said and picked up some of the wood.

Gideon chuckled. "Violet hates me choppin' wood, but she's to blame for gettin' me goin'. I was pretty worthless till she set me straight."

"Lit a fire under you, hmm? The Violet I knew was right quiet. She musta developed some a Lily's spunk."

"Yep." He grinned and grabbed a few of the smaller pieces. "But I sure as heck like it."

Caleb merely nodded. Their conversation got him thinking about Lily again and how much he appreciated her boldness and feisty spirit.

From what Gideon had said, her spunk had been badly doused. He prayed she'd gotten it back again.

As they neared the house, they were met with the scent of bacon.

Gideon sniffed the air. "Reckon you don't hafta cook this mornin'."

"You're right. I shoulda known my ma would see to it. We'll probably find her with Noah on one hip, Avery at her feet, an' a fork in one hand flippin' the bacon."

They laughed and went inside.

Caleb hadn't been far off. However, both children were seated at the table. Noah in the highchair, and Avery boosted up on pillows in a regular chair.

She grinned. "I big now."

"Yes, you are." He patted her head, then kissed her cheek.

"Pa!" Noah chirped and clapped his hands.

Avery giggled.

Caleb's ma looked over her shoulder from the stove, then rolled her eyes and shook her head. "Hope you boys are hungry."

"Yes'm," Gideon said. "Mind if I help myself to some a that there coffee?"

"I'll get it," Caleb said. "You go on an' sit down." He grabbed two mugs from the cupboard and filled them.

Gideon took the chair beside Noah. "Mornin', Noah." He placed a hand flat against the boy's forehead. "He don't feel hot no more. Violet's gonna be so relieved."

"Sissy."

"Yes, your sissy."

Caleb set the cups of coffee on the table and sat. "Do I smell cornbread, Ma?"

"Yep. It's almost done." She let out a huff. "You might need to check on Lucas. I ain't heard a peep from that room. He may a crawled out the window."

"The only way to get out that window would be to break it. It don't open, remember?"

"I plumb forgot." She speared the bacon and put it on a plate. "I woulda heard that for sure. You still best be checkin' on him."

Caleb took a quick sip of his coffee, then got up and headed down the hallway to the guestroom. He put his ear to the door. No sound whatsoever. Not even snoring.

He got the key and opened the door. "Lucas?"

Caleb crept close. Lucas was curled into a ball and wrapped tightly with the blankets. The entire mounded bundle shook.

"Lucas? You sick?"

"My head hurts," he rasped.

"You hungry?"

"No. Don't wanna eat nothin'. I just wanna sleep."

"All right." Caleb moved toward the door. "I'll leave this open. Yell if you need anythin'."

"Thanks, Caleb."

Thanks?

It had sounded heartfelt. Caleb cast a leery eye Lucas's way. The boy hadn't stopped shivering, and Caleb feared the worst.

He returned to the kitchen. "I got an awful feelin' Lucas has got the pox. Didn't see no blisters, but I think he's runnin' a fever. He's shiverin' an' buried 'neath the quilts."

His ma frowned. "You best leave him be. It'll hafta run its course."

He looked her in the eye. "What 'bout Becca an' Avery?" he whispered, not wanting his daughter to hear.

"Time will tell." She reached for a spoon and stirred a pot of oats.

"Oats *an'* cornbread?"

"Them oats is for Noah. To eat an' to bathe in. It'll help till I can get the calamine."

"Fine idea. Don't know why I didn't think of it." He sat down and grabbed his coffee. "Oh, an' Ma? When you go to town, can you send a telegram to Violet Myers in the cove? Gideon's agreed to stay a while to help, but wants her to know Noah's fine an' that

Lily's comin' to fetch him. But I reckon she might already know that. Even so, can you send the message?"

"Course. I gotta go by there anyways."

"To the telegram office? What for?"

His ma blinked rapidly and her mouth dropped open. "I meant, I gotta go by the hotel an' let Mrs. Iverson know what's goin' on, so she won't fret over me." She smiled a quirky grin, then stirred the pot again.

Caleb didn't press her for more information, but he knew without a doubt there was more to be said.

"Thank you for sendin' the telegram, Mrs. Henry," Gideon said. "My wife's with child, an' I don't want her worryin' herself an' upsettin' the baby. I've heard it can be hard on an unborn if their ma's troubled."

"Yes, it can. I'm happy to send the message."

"Thanks. An' when you see the doc, would you mind askin' him whether I need to be worried 'bout passin' on the pox from bein' 'round you all?"

"Don't mind at all. I planned to ask him if I'm contagious for the very same reason." She scooped some oats into a bowl, then poured a bit of cream on them and set them in front of Noah.

He stuck a finger in. "Hot."

Caleb scooted over beside him and blew on the cereal. "Can you hand me a spoon, Ma?"

She passed one over. Caleb dipped it in the oats, blew again, then tested them to make sure they were cool enough. "Mmm."

Like before, Noah imitated the sound.

Caleb spooned it into his mouth. If unborn children of expectant mothers were harmed from them being upset, had some kind of damage been done to this sweet boy?

He sure seemed good-natured. Unless Lucas was around, but that was understandable.

Avery pointed at Noah's cereal. "Mine?"

"Ma?" Caleb said. "Can you get a bowl for Avery?"

"Course I can." She patted the girl's head. "Sorry sweetheart. Gramma didn't mean to forget you."

Caleb had wondered if jealousy would become an issue for Avery. "Is Becca still sleepin'?"

"Yep. She was restless last night. I decided to fix breakfast an' leave her be."

Noah patted Caleb's hand. "More."

"Wanna do it yourself?" He handed Noah the spoon.

The boy fisted it and wiggled it into the cereal. A good deal went in his mouth, a lot more on his chin. But since his gramma was planning to bathe him in it, Caleb figured this was a good start.

A painful thought occurred to him. Caleb had been able to watch every stage of Avery's growth. And although Noah was still little, he'd missed a lot of his life. Even more painful was knowing that it had been taken away from Lily, too.

She'd been living in St. Louis and also in Asheville. Months had passed since she'd seen their son. Their reunion was long overdue.

However, the thought of seeing her both terrified and excited Caleb. He figured he had a couple more days to come up with the right words to say to her.

He hoped he wouldn't miserably fail.

Chapter 27

Lily perched next to Hiram on the buggy seat, but she couldn't be still. She rocked back and forth as if doing so would propel them faster.

"You're nervous as a jack rabbit," Hiram said. "I know you're worried 'bout your baby brother, but them little ones get over these kinda pox real well."

Lily sat tall and jutted her chin. "Noah's my son, not my brother."

"Oh." His head drew back. "No wonder you've been so beside yourself."

She gave him a sideways glance. "I shoulda told you sooner, but I didn't know what kind a man you was. I wanted to be sure you wouldn't go sayin' nasty things 'bout me to folks in Asheville. I may wanna go there again one day."

"I learned a long time ago not to judge folks." He clicked to the horses and got them moving faster.

"Thank you, Hiram."

"My pleasure, ma'am. I aim to keep prayin' that your boy is well."

She shut her eyes and did the same. The sound of a rider approaching opened them again. She studied his frame and realized he was missing a leg.

He brought the dapple gray horse close to the buggy. "Lily?"

"Gideon?" She'd not seen him in years, but there was no mistaking his handsome features. "What are you doin' all the way out here?"

Hiram pulled the buggy to a stop.

Gideon dipped his head. "I'm Gideon Myers, Miss Lily's brother-in-law."

Hiram returned a courteous nod, but Lily giggled. "Brother-in-law. I like the sound a that." She shook her head to regain her senses. "Now tell me. Why are you so far from home?"

"I came searchin' for Noah. When your pa told my pa 'bout Lucas runnin' off with the boy, Violet asked me to go after him. I didn't like the idea of ridin', but she convinced me I could do it. An' here I am."

"But you came from the other direction. You already been to Waynesville?"

"Yep. For a couple a days. Lucas told us he passed you headin' home to the cove. We all knew you'd come here once you seen Noah was gone. We figgered you wouldn't know how to find the Henry's place, so we all decided I should come lookin' for you to show you the way."

She waved her hands in the air. "We all? Who's we all?"

"Well, Caleb, his wife, Rebecca, an' his ma, Mrs. Henry."

She gaped at him, then snapped her mouth shut. "You sound like you've cozied up to them. Don't you find it a little odd?"

He moved his horse closer. "They're fine folks, Lily. An' Caleb has been takin' care a Noah like a good pa should."

She rubbed a hand over her heart. "So, they all know he's Noah's pa. Even his wife?"

"Yep, she does. I won't lie. She took it pretty hard, but considerin' the circumstances, I think she's handlin' it well. She's a good woman, but . . ."

"But what?" Tinges of jealousy crept in.

"She ain't never had the pox. Her daughter neither. They ain't showin' signs yet, but Lucas is bad off. His blisters just popped out an' he's runnin' a high fever. Caleb an' Mrs. Henry are tendin' him."

She turned to Hiram. "We gotta get movin'."

He rapidly nodded.

Lily waved her hand. "Gideon, show us the way."

He turned his horse around and kicked with his lone foot. The mare broke into a trot and they followed.

* * *

"Caleb." His ma grabbed him by the arm. "They're here."

He dropped onto the sofa and put his head in his hands. "I don't know if I'm ready for this."

"You?" She paced in front of the fireplace. "What 'bout me? I'm fixin' to meet your *Jezebel*."

He sat up straight. "Don't call her that. She's a fine woman." Now nervous for another reason, he stood and crossed to his ma. "Please, treat her kindly. She's been through hell."

"We all have." She rubbed her temples. "I'll behave. I promise. But I want you to know that I've never in my life been more uncomfortable."

"Imagine how Becca feels." He stared at the floor. "She's been dealin' with this incredibly well."

"That's because she's a fine an' decent woman. Exactly what I told you from the start. Remember that when you see Lily again, an' don't forget you're a married man."

"I won't. You can trust me on that."

Someone rapped on the front door and Caleb clutched his stomach. "Reckon Gideon felt the need to knock."

His ma shooed him toward the door. "Go on. The sooner we get this over with, the better."

Caleb's hand shook on the knob. He took several quick breaths and opened the door.

Gideon smiled in an odd sort of way and walked in. "I found 'em."

"Them?" Caleb drew his head back, then calmed. "Oh, that's right. She has a driver."

"He's gettin' her knapsack. Seems she plans to stay for a spell. An' since you're lackin' in beds, I best plan on leavin' soon."

Had Caleb heard him right? "Stayin'? For a spell?"

His ma rushed to them. "That won't do. It wouldn't be proper."

Gideon readjusted his crutch. "I understand, ma'am. But I told her 'bout Lucas bein' sick, an' she wants to help."

"We're tendin' him perfectly fine. She can't stay."

"Ma?" Caleb faced her straight on. "When she leaves, she'll take Noah with her. We're just gettin' to know him. I'd like to have as long as possible with my son. Don't you, too?"

She crossed her arms and grunted. "Yes. Maybe she can sleep in the barn."

"I'd never do that to her. We'll figger sumthin' out."

Gideon cleared his throat and nodded toward the front door.

Caleb spun around and nearly dropped to his knees. "Lily . . ." he whispered.

Nearly two years had passed since they'd stood face to face. Her hair was in disarray, poking out here and there from her braid, and her face was smudged with dirt.

She looked beautiful.

Their eyes locked and time reversed. Caleb's heart thumped harder with every second that passed.

"Hello, Caleb. It's been a while." She gulped and licked her lips.

She's as nervous as I am.

The man behind her squeezed in through the door. "I'm Hiram Baldwin. I've been watchin' over Miss Lily makin' certain she got where she needed to be. But I can't stay. I got a wife an' six kids I hafta get back to in Asheville."

Caleb forced his eyes from Lily and shook the man's hand. "Thank you. I appreciate what you done."

"Reckon I can fill up my canteen with water 'fore I head out?"

"Course you can," Caleb's ma said. "Come with me."

Caleb shook his head. She'd taken the easy way out and postponed introductions.

"I'll help," Gideon said and limped away.

Lily pushed the door shut. "It's a fine house, Caleb." She set her knapsack on the floor, then looked around the room as if she was trying to put her eyes on everything but him.

"Thank you. This is the where I grew up. I bought the farm from the folks what bought it from my ma." He pointed behind him. "That was her who took your driver for water. She's a mite nervous 'bout meetin' you."

Lily worked her lower lip with her teeth. "It's good to see you an' all, but where's Noah? I gotta see our boy. I'm achin' for him sumthin' fierce."

Caleb took two steps and lessened the space between them. "I understand." He took another step. "Lily, I—"

"The time will come for us to say what we need to. But it ain't now."

He longed to hold her and beg forgiveness for failing her, but as she said, it wasn't the right time. Besides, he had no right to hold her regardless of when it was.

"I'll fetch Noah. He's in my bedroom nappin'. Why don't you sit on the sofa? I'll bring him to you."

"Thank you."

She brushed past him on her way to sit down, pumping his blood faster.

If he didn't control his emotions, he'd make a bigger mess of this situation. He hurried down the hall, went to his room, and got their son.

Now came the hard part.

* * *

Lily pressed both hands to her heart, but it did no good. The heavy thumping reverberated in her ears. Nearly two years gone by, and Caleb looked better than ever.

It wasn't fair. Age and farm labor had made him into a full-fledged man.

Every feeling she'd tried to bury deep, bubbled to the surface. Her skin tingled and warmth filled her cheeks.

Don't do this to yourself. He's a married man.

She repeated the words over and over to herself. He wasn't hers and never would be.

"Lily?"

Even the way he said her name brought back pleasant memories.

She looked up and burst out crying. Sitting was no longer an option. She jumped to her feet and ran to her baby.

"Noah!"

Caleb passed him over and she clutched him against her pounding heart. Her love for her son exceeded all others.

"My Noah." She swayed with him in her arms. "I won't ever leave you again."

"Sissy." He patted her face, grinning.

Of course. It was the only way he knew her, but it felt like a knife to her heart.

"He doesn't know nothin' else," Caleb said. "Lucas told me Isaac an' Horace call you that. Noah calls every woman sissy. In time, he'll do what's right." Caleb placed a hand flat against Noah's back. "Won't you?"

Noah reached for him. "Pa."

"What? Why . . .?"

"Seems he calls every man pa."

"An' it looks like he wants you."

Noah kept stretching his arms toward Caleb, but she couldn't let him go.

Caleb motioned to the sofa. "Let's all sit. That might be easier."

None of this was easy, but she did as he suggested. She sat down and Caleb took the spot beside her. More memories flooded in.

Noah wiggled off her lap and onto his, then cuddled against his chest.

"I'm sorry, Lily. I've been tendin' him a couple a days now. He's gotten used to me. But given time, he'll bond with you. After all, you're his ma."

Noah lifted his head. "Ma."

"That's right, Noah. Lily ain't your sister, she's your ma."

"Sissy."

"No. *Ma.*" Caleb took Noah's tiny hand and touched it to Lily's arm. "Ma."

Noah giggled. "Ma."

Lily covered her mouth with her hand. "I ain't never heard him laugh like that before. It's the most beautiful sound." She closely examined his skin. "His pox is almost gone. He don't seem sick at all."

"He was half-naked an' runnin' a high fever when Lucas got him here. Becca cleaned him up good, an' when I came in I gave him a cool bath. Ma bathed him in oatmeal few days ago. That stopped the itchin'."

Lily tenderly rubbed Noah's back. "He coulda died in the woods. I never imagined Lucas could be so hateful an' do sumthin' that mean."

"You an' me both know Lucas is capable of many horrible things."

They were sitting so close, their breath mingled when they talked. Caleb's proximity sent her heart thumping again. "Gideon said he's bad off. I wanna stay here an' help, long as your wife is fine with that."

"Becca's restin' right now. She wants to meet you, Lily. She ain't bitter 'bout you an' me, but she don't like that I lied to her an' didn't tell her 'bout you." He ran his fingers along Noah's short tufts of hair. "Ma's havin' a harder time than anyone. She's fallen in love with Noah an' hates the thought a givin' him up."

Lily lifted her chin high. "Well, I can't stay here forever. I promised my pa I'd come back to the cove an' help him with the boys." She dropped her shoulders and shifted on the sofa to face him. "I'm sure Ma's dead by now. I made peace with her, but I could tell when I left, she didn't have much time."

Caleb set his hand on hers.

She startled, but didn't pull away.

He lightly rubbed across her skin. "I'm sorry 'bout your ma. I'm sorry 'bout *everythin'*."

Lily stared at their hands. His touch sent shivers down her spine and reached deep into her heart. They'd had something special together, and no matter what had happened between when they'd parted and now, she couldn't deny it. She still loved him.

"You must be Lily."

Lily whipped around and faced a beautiful young woman. Hair dark as night and defined facial features, though her cheeks were sunken. She looked half-starved.

"Yes, I'm Lily." She started to stand, but Rebecca motioned her down.

She sat gracefully in the seat across from them, crossed her ankles, and pulled them in. Her poise could have very well been taught by Mrs. Gottlieb. "I'm Rebecca. Caleb's wife."

"I'm happy to meet you," Lily said truthfully. "Thank you for carin' for my boy."

"Noah's precious. He an' my little Avery have grown fond of each other."

"She nappin'?"

"Yes." Rebecca folded her hands as if in prayer, but kept her head up. "How soon will you be leavin'?"

Lily opened her mouth to speak, but snapped it shut again, not knowing what to say.

Caleb cleared his throat. "She'd like to stay to tend her brother. At least till he's well enough to travel."

"That's right," Lily said. "Lucas can be a handful, but he doesn't scare me. My driver hasta get back to Asheville, but I reckon when the time comes for me to go, I'll hire a driver here in Waynesville to carry Lucas an' me home. An' Noah, of course."

"Of course." Rebecca smiled. She even *talked* proper.

Noah poked Lily in the arm. "Ma." He wriggled off Caleb's lap and moved onto hers. She thought she'd died and gone to Heaven.

She wrapped her arms around him and cuddled him close.

No one said another word.

Chapter 28

"I can't take this anymore!"

The yell broke the silence in the living room. Strangely welcome.

Lily craned her neck. "Was that Lucas?'

"Yep," Caleb said. "I'll go check on 'im."

"No. Let me." Lily passed Noah into Caleb's arms. "I need to have a heart to heart with my brother."

Rebecca's brows drew together. "But he's sick. It might not be the right time to talk to him 'bout serious matters."

Lily stood and smoothed her skirt. "Actually, it's the perfect time. He's too weak to be unmanageable."

"That's a very good point." Rebecca smiled a genuine smile. "It's the last room on the left."

"I'm sure I can find it. I'll just follow the moans." She headed down the hallway.

The bedroom smelled far from pretty. She couldn't expect Rebecca or Mrs. Henry to clean up after him, but Lily certainly would. He needed his bedding changed and a clean nightshirt.

Lucas himself wasn't pretty either. He violently scratched at his sores.

"You keep that up an' they'll get infected." Lily sat in a chair beside the bed. "Wanna be scarred the rest a your life?"

"Lily? When did you get here?"

"A short while ago." She crossed her arms and glared at him. "Why'd you try to kill my boy?"

Lucas grunted. "I don't wanna talk to you."

"You don't have a choice. If you tell me all I wanna know, I might be kind enough to make some medicine that'll do much better than calamine. I made some for Isaac an' Horace an' it worked real good."

He clawed at his arm. "I just want it to stop."

"Fine. So tell me. Why'd you wanna kill Noah?"

"I didn't. I only wanted him outta our house. Away from Ma."

She leaned close. "So you hauled him through the mountains only half-dressed while he was sufferin' a fever an' pox?" She breathed hard and heavy. "That ain't no way to treat a baby!"

"Sorry." He scowled. "Reckon my mind wasn't right at the time. I was mad cuz Ma was dyin'. An' it was Noah's fault. If he hadn't given her the pox, she'd be fine now."

"An' if Ma hadn't sent Noah to the Hendersons, they'd all be fine. So whose fault is it truly? Hmm?"

Lucas's mouth screwed together. He sat up and scratched his legs, then leaned way down and dug his nails between his toes. "Make me that medicine, Lily, or this is gonna kill me."

"You keep scratchin' an' it might. I ain't lyin', Lucas. Them sores get infected, an' it won't be good." She looked into his green eyes and saw something she'd never seen before.

Fear.

Compassion took hold of her. She brushed her hand across the top of his head. "I'll go gather what I need for the medicine. I'm sure I can find a white oak 'round here somewhere."

"Thank you, Lily. I mean it."

She believed him.

* * *

"She's nice," Rebecca whispered and meant it. "Pretty, too." She watched to see her husband's reaction.

He appeared so comfortable on the sofa with Noah on his lap. The two had bonded, and Rebecca knew Caleb would have difficulty letting his son go. Not to mention, she'd seen the way Caleb had looked at Lily. He'd never looked at her that way.

"Yes, she is," Caleb finally said. It had taken him a while to respond. He probably feared saying something that might upset her.

Lately, everything had bothered her. Yet any stranger on the outside peering in would agree that she had every right to be troubled. But having the right didn't make her feel any better.

"Where do we go from here, Caleb?"

His eyes focused on the boy. "I thought you said you was movin' to the hotel?"

"Honestly, I don't want to. An' I know it'll upset Avery bein' away from you. But how can I stay here as your wife, when I know you'd rather be with Lily?"

"Becca. Don't say that."

"But it's true. An' I can see why. She's lovely. An' unlike me, she's strong."

He lifted his head. "You just met her. How can you tell she's strong?"

"She traveled a long way to get to Noah. That alone requires strength. But I also saw it in her actions here." A little laugh escaped her. "What she said 'bout Lucas."

"You're strong in other ways, Becca. You're a wonderful ma." He grinned. "An' you make a great pie."

"I think that's what got you an' me in trouble. My pies won you over, but I didn't capture your heart."

"That's not true." He repositioned Noah and scooted to the edge of the sofa. "We swore we'd tell each other the truth from here on out. You've been in my heart since we was kids."

"An' you've been in mine. But for me, I see you as a lover. I think you love me as a sister. Someone who's part of your family. I know you care 'bout me, but it's not the same. An' it's not the kind a love I need from a husband."

"But—"

"Don't, Caleb. It's all right. I've accepted it. Least I know that I'm not crazy. As for what we should do . . ." She looked downward and let out a breath. "I don't know yet. Let's give it a little time an' we'll figure it out."

She glanced toward the window. "It's a beautiful day. I think I'll get Avery an' take her outside to swing." She stood and moved toward the hallway.

Caleb didn't budge from the couch. She knew she'd given her husband plenty to think about.

* * *

Lily rushed out the front door, though she was tempted to sit down beside Caleb again. But since she'd promised medicine for Lucas, she had to set those thoughts aside.

She spotted Gideon heading toward the barn and hurried after him.

It didn't take her long to catch up with him. "You gettin' ready to leave?"

"Yep. I feel better goin' home now that the doc confirmed I won't pass anythin' on to Violet. Anythin' special you want me to tell her?"

"Just let her know I love her, an' that I'll be home as soon as I can. An' tell her, I don't aim to leave the cove ever again."

He beamed. "Promise to hurry up, so you can be there when our baby's born."

"When's it due?"

"Middle a July."

They walked into the barn and he motioned to a saddle draped over one of the stall slats. "Reckon you can help me saddle up Stardust?"

"I'm happy to."

"Good. We gotta wrangle her up first. She might not like leavin'." They went back outside and scanned the field. She was some distance away.

Lily shielded her eyes from the sun. "She's a beauty. Where'd you get her?"

"Your pa. She was his, then he gave her to us as a weddin' gift."

Lily sighed. "I wish I'd been there." She spotted a lead draped over the fence and grabbed it. "I'll go fetch her. You wait here, then we'll saddle her together."

"Thank you. She's real gentle. Shouldn't give you any trouble."

Lily ran into the field. Caleb certainly had a nice place. She counted at least five other horses and a dozen cattle. He had to be doing quite well financially.

"Stardust!"

The mare tossed her head.

"Time to go, girl." Lily eased up next to her and put the lead over her head. She didn't fight, but nosed around Lily as if searching for something. "They been givin' you treats?"

The horse didn't answer. Good thing, too.

Lily led her back to Gideon. "You got enough food to get you by till you're home?"

"Yep. Mrs. Henry packed up some biscuits, jerky, and even some a her preserves. I should be fine."

They headed for the stall and Lily grabbed the saddle. She hoisted it atop the mare and Gideon helped strap it down.

"Lily?"

His tone sounded serious.

"Sumthin' wrong?"

He leaned against the railing. "Caleb's a good man. I've gotten to know him, an' I like him. He loves Noah, so . . . try an' work sumthin' out so he can see him now an' then. All right?"

"I'm glad you got to know him. Maybe you can tell Violet that he's not the vile beast she thinks he is."

He laughed. "I will."

"As for workin' sumthin' out." She chewed at her lip. "I don't know how. It ain't easy bein' three days apart. But I promise, if he comes to the cove to see Noah, I won't be hateful."

Gideon stroked Stardust's nose. "You still love him, don't you?"

"Does it matter?"

Gideon shook his head, then fastened his crutch into a strap at Stardust's side. He put his foot in the stirrup and mounted. "Not bad for a one-legged man, huh?"

"I'm impressed." She grinned. "You grew up fine, Gideon Myers. I used to think you were a little stinker. Glad you grew out of that."

"Oh, I can be a stinker if I wanna be. Just ask Violet."

"I will." She reached up and took his hand. "Take care a yourself goin' home. My sister needs you." She squeezed and released him. "Ain't you gonna tell everyone else goodbye?"

"Already have. While you was fussin' at Lucas." Gideon snickered.

"Lucas! I nearly forgot the white oak. That boy will be scratched up to high heaven." She rushed from the barn with Gideon following her.

"Bye, Lily!" He clicked to the horse.

"Bye! See you soon!"

She watched him ride away, then spotted a white oak not far from her. Time to make medicine.

She was surprised that Hiram hadn't told her goodbye before *he'd* left. Seemed he'd gotten his canteen filled and left without another word. He probably saw that she was tied up in conversation and didn't want to disturb her. Besides, he'd said he had to get home to his family. She couldn't fault him for that.

She'd be sure to write him a letter of thanks.

While plucking a few leaves from the tree and scraping some bark, she swore she heard singing. Once she'd gotten the ingredients for the medicine, she followed the sound. Sure enough, she found Rebecca with her little girl. They were on a swing suspended from a thick tree branch.

"That looks like fun," Lily said, laughing.

"Wee!" the child yelled.

If Lily's memory served her well, the girl's name was Avery.

Rebecca brought the swing to a halt. "What have you got there?" She nodded to the leaves in Lily's hand.

"I'm gonna fix some medicine for Lucas. White oak leaves an' bark steeped together help relieve itchin'."

"Truly?" Rebecca's head tipped to the side. "Where did you learn that?"

"My ma. We learned all kinds of ways to make medicine from nature. The Cherokee Indians passed on their knowledge."

Avery hopped from her ma's lap and pointed at Lily, questioning with her eyes.

Rebecca smiled. "This is Miss Lily. She's Noah's ma."

Lily squatted down in front of the girl. "An' what's your name?"

"Avey."

Rebecca laughed. "She has trouble with her r's."

Lily smiled at the child. "That's a lovely name. You like the swing, don't you?"

She nodded. "You swing."

"Me?" Lily eyed the temptation. "Only for a second, then I gotta go cook up some medicine."

Lily set the leaves and bark on the ground, then sat on the swing. Before she could get it going, Avery climbed into her lap. Lily held onto the girl and kicked off.

She closed her eyes and let the wind dust her face. "No wonder you like this. I do, too."

Lily glanced over at Rebecca who was studying them closely. Lily hoped she hadn't overstepped her bounds. She stopped the swing, helped Avery off, then stood and scooped up her things from the ground.

"She's a sweet girl," Lily said.

"Yes, she is." Rebecca fidgeted with the front of her dress. "You're good with children. Gideon said you were workin' as a nanny in Asheville. I'm sure they miss you."

"I miss them, too. But they wanted me to be with Noah. They understood."

"Will you go back to Asheville, or home to the cove?"

"I gotta go home. They need me more than the folks in Asheville. But someday, I wanna go visit them again. I got attached." She smiled, thinking of little Levi. "I really love children."

"I'm glad."

Avery tugged at her ma's hand and led her back to the swing.

Lily pondered Rebecca's remark. It seemed odd. Yet she probably meant she was glad for Noah's sake. Or maybe she was just happy to know that Lily wasn't a hateful person. It might make it easier for her to understand how Caleb could've fallen in love with her.

And though Lily had sometimes doubted that he had, she no longer did. Not after the way he'd looked at her when she'd walked into his home.

The sooner she left, the better it would be for Rebecca and him.

She returned to the house and went in the back entrance that led to the kitchen. She nearly hit Mrs. Henry with the door.

The woman squealed.

"I'm so sorry," Lily said, clutching onto the items from the tree. "You must be Caleb's ma."

"An' you must be Lily." She eyed her up and down. "I'd say it's good to finally meet you, but I don't like to lie."

Her words were a heavy blow. "I'm sorry you feel that way, ma'am." She swallowed the lump in her throat and motioned to the stove. "Mind if I cook up some medicine for my brother?"

"That's fine. There's pots over yonder." No smile and very matter-of-fact.

Caleb had said his ma was nervous about meeting her, but she didn't seem that way at all. She was the first person to be hateful to Lily since her arrival. Even Lucas was nicer. Well—after she'd threatened him.

Lily found an appropriate pot, then dumped in some water from a pitcher on the counter. She put the ingredients in the pan, then set it on the stove. "It's just gotta heat up an' steep a bit."

"Make sure the children don't get into it."

"Oh, I'm real careful 'round little ones. Rest assured."

Mrs. Henry took a seat at the kitchen table. "I love my daughter-in-law. I don't wanna see her hurt."

Lily also sat. "I'd never wanna hurt her. She's kind."

"Your presence alone makes it difficult for her. An' Avery has been confused since your brother showed up." She thrummed her fingers on the table.

"Ma'am." Lily took a large breath. "I know we've disrupted your lives, an' I'm truly sorry for that. But none of this was intentional." Tears were forming and Lily wished she could stop them. "Love does things sometimes that hurt. I promise, as soon as my brother's well, we'll leave. But I'm takin' Noah with me. He's my son, an' I love him more than anythin'."

"He's Caleb's son, too." Mrs. Henry firmed her jaw. "An' my grandson."

"I'm well aware. But I ain't gonna leave him here. That's not an option. You can come visit whenever you please, but I won't leave him behind."

Mrs. Henry blinked and a tear dropped onto her cheek.

The woman had a heart. "You've grown fond a my boy, haven't you?"

"Yes. He's so much like Caleb when he was a baby. It's like steppin' back in time. An' he's so sweet."

Lily scooted her chair over and took her hand.

The woman's eyes grew wide, but she didn't pull away.

"Mrs. Henry, your son meant the world to me. I don't know how much he told you 'bout me an' our situation, but I swear to you, Noah was conceived in love. This is hard on all of us, but we gotta make it work. Somehow." Lily swiped at her own tears.

Mrs. Henry looked straight at her. "Forgive me for bein' hateful. I wanted to dislike you. An' I'd hoped you'd be a poor ma, so I'd have good reason to keep Noah here. But why would I ever think my son would fall in love with a horrid woman? I shoulda known better."

"He told you he was in love with me?"

"Yes. An' I see now I was wrong to dissuade him. Reckon we've all learned from this." She fingered Lily's hair. "It's a nice color, but it could use a good brushin', an' maybe a washin'."

Lily pulled a strand forward. "I ain't seen my reflection in a mirror for days. I must be a sight."

Mrs. Henry cupped Lily's cheek. "You're still a pretty girl." She nodded toward the stove. "Your medicine is boilin'."

Lily jumped up and moved the pot from the heat. "Now it's gotta set a short while, an' I can go doctor Lucas."

"I'll find some fresh blankets for you to use on the sofa. Gideon said it slept pretty well, so I hope you'll be comfortable."

"Thank you, ma'am."

Mrs. Henry donned a sad smile. "Stay as long as you hafta." She got up and left the kitchen.

Lily looked out the window at the blue sky. "Ma, if you're up there, send an angel to help us here. We're gonna need it."

Chapter 29

Lily shut Lucas's door as quietly as possible. They no longer locked it, because he'd grown too weak to get out of bed. Lily had ended up tending him much in the same manner in which she'd cared for Arabelle.

Lucas didn't complain about her care and accepted it without question. But Lily was certain he was a little embarrassed by it all.

The medicine she'd made—along with a few oatmeal baths—had stopped the itching, but it sounded as if the illness had moved into his lungs. It wasn't anywhere close to the severity, but if Lily didn't do something soon, it could become similar to that of their ma.

If only Lily had arrived in the cove sooner, she might've been able to save her.

Though Lily was no doctor, the remedies her ma had taught her for treating most any ailment always seemed to work. Maybe her pa had tried using a poultice, but she doubted he'd attempted. He'd never been able to recall exact ingredients.

She went to the kitchen and walked in on Caleb and Rebecca, sitting at the table talking. They stopped the instant she appeared.

"Sorry," she said. "I didn't mean to interrupt."

"You're fine," Rebecca said. "We weren't discussin' anythin' of importance."

Lily had been there four days. They'd established a daily routine and everyone behaved amicably, but she still felt like an intruder. "Do you have any onions?"

Rebecca nodded. "They're in the root cellar."

Caleb grinned. "Are *you* cookin' supper t'night?"

"No. I need them for Lucas. I gotta make a poultice to relieve his lungs. He's started to breathe poorly, an' I wanna clear it up 'fore it gets too bad."

Caleb stood, shaking his head and smiling. "You shoulda gone to medical school, Lily. You probably coulda taught *them* sumthin'. You wait right here, I'll get the onions. How many do you need?"

"Two good-sized ones."

He nodded and left.

Rebecca patted the seat beside her. "Sit down. You look tired."

"I am. Takin' care a Lucas has me spent." She plopped into the chair, then laid her head on the table. "I'm glad Mrs. Henry is tendin' Noah right now."

"She has Avery, too." Rebecca softly laughed. "My mother-in-law loves bein' a gramma."

Lily rose up and examined Rebecca's face. "You sure you feel all right? No aches in your head? Fever? Itchy skin?"

"Stop worryin' 'bout me. I feel no different than I normally do. It's been a week since Lucas came. I'm sure I won't get sick."

Lily prayed she was right, but the doctor had told Mrs. Henry that it sometimes took up to two weeks before symptoms showed.

"Here you are." Caleb extended two large onions. "Will these do?"

"Perfect." Lily found the energy to get on her feet, grab the onions, and get a frying pan. "I also need a soft cloth for the poultice. Do you have sumthin' you don't mind stinkin' up with onion?"

Caleb glanced at Rebecca, then returned his attention to Lily. "We can use one a Avery's old diapers. It's clean, an' it's been stunk up before."

"That'll work." Lily set the frying pan on the stove and heated a bit of water in it. She quickly sliced the onions and threw them in.

Caleb came back with the diaper and set it on the counter. "You sure that's not supper? It smells mighty good."

"They do taste good this way, but Lucas needs 'em. If you want, I can cook some more up later fried in lard, not water. Then, they're real tasty." She stirred the onion around till it was soft, but not brown.

"My eyes are waterin' all the way over here," Rebecca said. "Those are some potent onions."

"An' that's a good thing," Lily said. "Well, not that your eyes are waterin', but the more potent the onions, the better they work." She removed the pan from the heat, then carefully drained off the water and set the onions aside.

The size of the old diaper was just right. She smoothed it out, then spread the onions in the center. "Now all I gotta do is fold this up an' put it on Lucas's chest. He should start coughin' up all the crud in no time."

"Lily?" Rebecca got up from her chair and peered over Lily's shoulder.

"Yes?"

"If I *do* get sick, I hope you'll still be here to tend me." She timidly smiled, then slowly walked out of the kitchen.

Lily looked over at Caleb. "There sumthin' I should know?"

His brows crinkled. "She ain't been eatin' right for some time now, an' she has slowed down quite a bit."

"Don't she have an appetite?"

"No. She said once, that she don't enjoy food no more." He turned away. "I admit, I'm worried 'bout her."

Lily lightly patted his back, then thought better of it and pulled her hand to herself. "If she truly wants me near, I'll stay long enough to make sure she's all right. An' if it comes down to it, I'll look after her."

He shifted around and faced her. "Thank you, Lily."

She picked up the poultice. "Remind you of anythin'?"

"Yep. But mine didn't stink."

Being near him this way was never easy. She'd been trying all she could to avoid time alone with him.

She gestured to his shoulder. "How's that wound?"

Caleb had been smiling and almost playful, but his expression became solemn and somewhat sad. He tapped the spot. "That one's fine. It's this one that hasn't healed." He put his hand over his heart.

She swallowed hard, then hurried down the hall to Lucas's room.

Caleb had to know the effect he had on her. But their situation was hopeless, and they simply had to get over it.

At least tending Lucas would get her mind off the past she and Caleb shared.

The scent from the onions stung her eyes, but she was grateful for their potency.

"Lucas?"

He didn't stir.

She set the poultice on top of the bureau, then moved to the bed. Lucas was lying on his side, so she pulled the blankets off and eased him onto his back. She unbuttoned his nightshirt and bared his chest. The onion might irritate the sores, but it was more important to rid his lungs of congestion.

She laid the poultice on his skin. "Breathe deep as you can, Lucas."

He moaned. His eyes fluttered open, but stayed half shut. "What's that smell?"

"It's onion. I made you a poultice. You got a lotta crud in your lungs that hasta come out. This should make you cough." She sat in the chair beside him, then put her hand to his head. "You're still burnin' up. I'll get a cool cloth for your forehead."

She started to rise, but he held out a hand. "Wait."

"What's wrong?"

"Why are you bein' so nice to me?" He spoke so quietly, nothing like his normal self. Yet his illness likely kept the strength from his voice.

"Lucas, don't try an' talk. Just breathe in that onion."

He inhaled a few times and sputtered a bit, but nowhere close to what he needed to do.

"Lily, I got things I hafta say."

"Whatever it is, it can wait. When you get better—"

"After what I done to Noah, why don't you let me die?"

She took hold of his hand. "Don't say that. Even with all we've been through, an' all the times I haven't liked you much, you're still my brother. I love you, Lucas."

She looked into his face and swore his eyes had filled with tears.

He turned his head.

"Lucas? When you was little, you got real sick an' Ma fixed a poultice just like this one. I remember bein' so scared that we was gonna lose you. But you had a few coughin' fits an' got better. I know you will again."

He coughed. A stronger one this time.

She squeezed his hand. "Remember when we used to climb trees together? You always had to go higher than me—just to prove yourself. You was happy then. We all were."

"That was 'fore the war," he mumbled. "I was only nine when it started. An' the first time soldiers came to our cabin, I was so scared I wet myself." He hacked real hard, then frowned and looked down. "I ain't never told anyone that. I reckon Ma knew since she washed my things. But I decided I was gonna prove I could be a man an' stand up to anyone. So I got tough."

His coughing had jostled the poultice, so she firmed it back in place. "There was no need for you to toughen up then. You was *only* nine. You wasn't expected to act like a man. We was all scared, but we got through it. Course, it was hardest on Pa."

Lucas's chin vibrated. "Don't talk 'bout Pa." He breathed heavily, then coughed up some phlegm and spit it on the floor.

Lily grabbed a bucket she'd brought in for potential vomit and set it next to him. "Use this next time." She sat back down. It appeared as if Lucas was about to cry outright, and it would only make him weaker. "You should try to calm down. Bein' upset ain't good for healin'."

A single sob erupted from him. "I put lye in Pa's moonshine."

"Do what?" She gaped at him. "Are you confessin' all your sins thinkin' you're gonna die, or do you want me to hate you?"

"Just let me die, Lily. I'm tired a livin'." He coughed, cried, and coughed some more.

"You're only fifteen years old, Lucas Larsen. Too young to die. Get yourself right an' you might find that life's worth livin'." She stood and headed for the door. "I need some air. I'll be back to check on you later."

She walked out without waiting for a response. The good Lord could forgive any sin, but Lily was human. Though she loved her brother, forgiving him would take a great deal of work, as well as Lucas showing proof that he deserved it.

Chapter 30

Lily flipped around and faced the back of the sofa. It had been comfortable the first few nights, but she missed sleeping on a real bed.

The others in the house were already stirring. She needed to get up and check on Noah, but it was a bit awkward since he slept with Caleb. It wouldn't be pleasant when the time came to break their bond.

Someone knocked on the front door, and she popped her head up.

She groaned and sat completely up, then raked her fingers through her tousled hair.

Caleb walked in holding Noah. "Did I hear someone knock?"

She nodded and yawned.

"Ma." Noah reached for her. He'd been calling her that since the day on the sofa when Caleb had set him straight. She'd never tire of hearing it.

Caleb passed him to her. "You might not wanna be seen right now. Hard to say who's at the door."

"Do I look that bad, or are you afraid what folks might say if they find out I'm here? You know—gossip an' all."

"Maybe a little a both." He cast a quirky grin. "But seriously, Lily, whoever's here must not know we got pox in the house. If they knew, they'd keep their distance."

Another knock.

"Better answer it," she said. "I'll take Noah an' go to the kitchen."

She walked away, but hid herself around the corner, so she could listen.

"Ma," Noah patted her face.

"Shh." She kissed his cheek and moved him to her other hip, farther away from view.

They'd had another visitor two days prior. A messenger who'd brought a telegram from Violet. Gideon had arrived home safely, and all was well with them, but as Lily feared, her ma had passed.

Maybe it was another messenger.

The door squeaked open.

"Hello, Caleb."

There was no mistaking the voice of Vincent Douglas.

She marched into the living room. "What are you doin' here?"

"I should ask the same of you, Lily. As always, it's a pleasure to see you. Though I must say you've let yourself go." He smirked and casually folded his hands in front of himself.

Caleb stepped between them. "Why *are* you here? Are you aware there are folks with chickenpox in this house?"

Vincent calmly kept his stance. "Yes. But I'm only interested in one person in particular. I received a telegram from your mother. She said that Callie had returned and was staying here. I've come to collect her."

"What?" Caleb stared at the man, then turned, wide-eyed, to Lily.

"Callie ain't here," she quickly said. "Seems you came a long way for nothin'." She lightly bounced Noah in her arms.

Vincent eyed him, then Caleb. "May I please enter? Instinct tells me there's more going on here than I expected to find. I can see the boy had the pox, but he looks quite well. I've had them before, so I'm not concerned about becoming ill. However, I intend to get to the bottom of this. If the telegram was meant to mislead me—"

"It wasn't."

Lily turned to find Rebecca standing behind her. Mrs. Henry stood farther away holding Avery.

Rebecca's face was pale and her steps were slow, but deliberate. She pushed past Lily and faced Vincent. "I asked my mother-in-law to send the telegram. Come inside an' we'll talk 'bout it." She stepped back and motioned him in.

"Becca?" Caleb questioned her with his eyes, but she sadly shook her head.

Lily rushed to the sofa and moved the blanket that had covered her. Noah clung onto a corner of it, so she sat in a chair and let him cuddle it. Her heart thumped hard. Why had Rebecca sent for the man?

Vincent casually sat on the sofa. His prideful air churned Lily's stomach.

Silence fell over the room as everyone took a seat.

Rebecca twisted her fingers together. "I did what I thought I needed to at the time."

Vincent crossed his legs and eased back against the cushions. "Are you saying you changed your mind and let Callie go?"

"No. There is no Callie."

Lily exchanged looks with Caleb, but they both remained quiet. If he felt anything like her, he'd be wondering how this would play out.

His ma just sat there with Avery, appearing both at ease and uncomfortable. A hard thing to do.

Vincent leaned forward. "Don't toy with me. I've traveled too far to play games."

Rebecca sat tall. "My husband was in the cove at the time of the shootin'. He dressed like a woman so folks there wouldn't know the Larsens had a man in their home."

Lily wanted to shrink into the floor. Why was Rebecca doing this?

Vincent grunted a laugh and gave Caleb a sideways smirk. "So, *you* were Callie?"

"Yes." He pulled his shoulders back. "But I didn't kill Ableman."

"Of course you did. I saw you holding the gun. But for the life of me I can't understand why your lovely wife would want to turn you over to me. You'll likely be hung."

"But he didn't shoot 'im!" Lily blurted out. "He's tellin' you the truth!"

Vincent cocked his head. "Did you?"

Lily drew Noah closer, simply to feel a secure presence. "No," she whispered.

How could she tell the truth? Lucas had saved her from Ableman and kept Caleb from being killed.

"Then, who did?" Vincent looked from face to face.

Rebecca stood and crossed to Lily. "I'm so sorry." She turned toward Vincent. "As I said, when I asked for the telegram to be sent, I thought I was doin' right. After all, the boy had been hateful an' mean. I feared for my family."

"What boy?"

Rebecca's hand shook. She braced herself against the sofa. "Lucas Larsen." Her knees buckled and she crumbled to the floor.

"Becca!" Caleb jumped to his feet and lifted her into his arms. "She's on fire." He rushed down the hall, cradling Rebecca's limp body.

Lily got up to follow him, but stopped when Avery burst out bawling. Mrs. Henry swayed with her, yet couldn't ease her.

Lily stroked the girl's hair. "Let's take the children to Avery's room. Then I'll check on Rebecca."

"Ma!" Avery cried.

"Your ma will be fine." Lily kissed her cheek, finding it warmer than usual. "I think she's comin' down with it, too."

Mrs. Henry hurried away.

"Wait one minute!" Vincent stood erect. "What does Lucas have to do with all this? The last I knew, he'd gone home to a dying mother."

Lily moved within inches of him, glaring. Noah clung onto her. "Our ma did die. Lucas came here an' brought the pox with him. He's in the room down the hall likely dyin' himself." She peered into his eyes, no longer afraid. "*He* shot Ableman. That poor excuse for a man wanted me. Callie, too. An' you know darn well what I mean. If not for Lucas, Ableman woulda had me. Probably after killin' Caleb, once he found out he wasn't no girl. So who's in the wrong here? Hmm?"

"I took your brother into my care. I believed him about Callie, yet he knew all this time we were searching for someone nonexistent. He played me."

"An' you played Mrs. Ableman. You spent her money mostly on women. Ain't that right? You taught my brother to be despicable like you and how to fool folks into believin' you were respectable. He was fourteen. Nowhere close to bein' a man. He needed guidance, but you ruined him."

"Lucas enjoyed every moment." He stuck his nose high in the air. "If he doesn't die, I'll have him imprisoned. Not only for murder, but for deceiving me and Mrs. Ableman. She's a good woman who didn't deserve to be misled."

"An' what will that good woman think when I let her know how her money was spent? Not only by you, but by the boy you corrupted. I know folks who could back up my story."

"Who? Your brother?" He laughed. "He's lied about everything else, she wouldn't believe him in that regard. She respects me."

"I have friends in St. Louis. They run a home for wayward women called Waters Rest. The women there know all that goes on in them steamboats on the river. A man like you would be hard to forget."

Another laugh. "Mrs. Ableman would *not* entertain testimony from prostitutes."

"I never said they was prostitutes." Lily took a step back, but kept her eyes glued to his. "I have a suggestion for you. Go back to St. Louis an' tell your employer that when you got here you found out Callie had died from the pox. Your work would be done."

"Why should I? Justice should be served."

Her throat tightened. "Tell that to my brother. The boy you tainted. Was it justice to corrupt a child? If he gets well, I aim to do all I can to get him right again. I know his good heart is in there somewhere."

Vincent turned his steely eyes to Noah. "Is this your child, Lily?"

"Yes." She jutted her chin.

"Then tell me, who here is truly tainted?" He spun on his heels and marched to the door, then paused and looked over his shoulder. "You won't see me again." He walked out and slammed the door shut.

Lily jumped and Noah's arms flailed.

"It's all right, baby. The bad man is gone."

Even so, she faced something much worse.

She breathed deeply and carried Noah to Avery's room, where she found Mrs. Henry perched on the edge of the child's bed.

"I heard every word," she said. Her brows dipped in worry, and she kept her eyes on Avery. "You're a brave woman, Lily. You can be proud of what you said." She sniffled and rubbed the child's little hand. "What are we gonna do? I prayed this wouldn't happen, but feared it would."

Lily set Noah down. He headed for Avery's toys.

"We're gonna take care a them, just like we done for Lucas an' Noah. An' they'll be fine."

Mrs. Henry lifted her head. "But Rebecca hasn't been well—even before this happened. She's undernourished. How can she fight this illness?"

"She'll hafta give it her all. An' I'll do what I can to help her." Lily nodded toward Noah. "Mind watchin' him? I wanna look in on Rebecca. Lucas, too."

"You go on. I'll see to the children."

Lily bent down and hugged her. "Keep them prayers comin'." She squeezed a bit tighter, then released her and walked away.

* * *

This couldn't be happening.

Caleb gently placed Rebecca on their bed, then covered her with two quilts. "Warm enough?"

She shivered. "Can you lay down with me an' put your arms 'round me?"

"Course I can." He lay atop the blankets, drew her close, then made sure the quilts were firmly tucked around her back.

She rested her head on his chest. "I'm scared, Caleb. Everythin' hurts."

He placed a soft kiss on the top of her head, amazed at the amount of heat that emanated from her body. "You don't hafta be afraid. I'm here, an' Lily promised to take care a you, too. You'll get better so don't fret."

She tipped her head back and looked up at him. "Lily's a good woman. If sumthin' happens to me—"

"Hush. I don't want you talkin' like that. You should sleep. It's best when you're sick."

"Will you stay with me? Least for a little while?"

"Yes. I won't go nowhere." He rubbed her back, trying to ease her into sleep. Soon, the pocks would come out and she'd no longer care to be touched.

Lily appeared in the doorway. She cast a sad smile, then nodded and walked off.

His mind tumbled with too many thoughts. Loving two women hadn't been smart. Worse yet, he couldn't bear the idea of losing either one of them.

Chapter 31

The scent of sizzling onions filled the kitchen.

Lily stirred them around, then drained them and prepared another poultice. Lucas had improved, but needed another treatment.

As for Rebecca, she was in the early stages of the pox. Her blisters had just formed and they were using every means available to keep the irritation down. They did the same for Avery. The poor little girl fussed, not understanding her condition. Her gramma continuously stayed by her side.

Noah wandered between Lily and Caleb, vying for attention. Now that Noah was well, he sometimes entertained himself, but still liked to cling. Lily wished things were different so she could solely focus on him. But not yet . . .

"I know you don't like the smell, Lucas, but it's helpin'." Lily set the poultice on his chest.

"Why can't you make it outta sumthin' good-smellin'? Like flowers?"

"Flowers won't make you hack up that crud." She sat primly straight. "Now, breathe deep and get to coughin'." She placed the bucket beside him.

"I'll never eat another onion." He hacked and spit.

"Least you're talkin' 'bout eatin'. That's a good sign."

His mouth twisted from side to side, then he huffed a breath. "Thank you for not givin' up on me. I know how mad you was. An' you had every right to be."

"That I did." She dropped her shoulders and contemplated how to say things right. All the things Mr. Jacobson had told her about his sister and family came to mind. "Sometimes, folks ain't given a second chance. What if I told you that you could start over from scratch? As if you'd never done a thing wrong?"

"I thought only Jesus could do that."

She laughed. Maybe he had learned something in church. "I ain't Jesus, but I know sumthin' you don't."

"Oh?" He scooted higher in the bed. The poultice slipped, but he put it back in place.

"Yep. When you was delirious, Vincent Douglas came callin'."

Lucas's eyes grew wide. "He was here? What for?"

"Rebecca sent for him. Claimed she had Callie here."

"That don't make no sense." He'd gotten a little too loud.

Lily touched a finger to her lips. "Rebecca is sleepin', so keep your voice down."

"Fine. Now tell me. Why'd she do that?"

"She thought you was gonna hurt her family, but she came to realize you wouldn't. By then it was too late. She told him Caleb was Callie, then I told him you were the one who shot Ableman."

Lucas scowled and his body deflated. "I thought you was tryin' to help me."

"I did. The truth is out. You don't have anythin' to hide from. I convinced Vincent to tell Mrs. Ableman that Callie died from pox."

"An' he agreed?" His expression softened.

"Yep. I can be persuasive when I wanna be." She took his hand. "He won't bother us again, but you hafta promise me sumthin'."

"What?"

"I want you to come home with me an' Noah. Ma's gone, an' Pa's gonna need us."

"But what 'bout the lye in his moonshine? He'll never trust me again."

"He doesn't hafta know. You made a mistake an' I believe you're sorry for it." She sat back in her chair. "You'll hafta help with the farm. I know you hate it, but like I said, Pa needs us."

"I don't really hate it. I just always knew I could never measure up to you."

She shook her head. "We're different from each other, but I'm no better than you. We all make mistakes." She sat tall once again. "So, will you go with me?"

He smiled. "I'd like that."

"One more thing."

His eyes narrowed. "What?"

"If you ever lay a hand on Noah again, I swear I'll turn you over my knee an' whup your hide. Understood?"

He snickered. "You ain't been able to do that since I was eight."

"I'm stronger now." She pointed a finger in his face. "Don't push it." Grinning, she got to her feet. "I'm gonna make you some broth. No onions."

She'd never believed it could happen, but she honestly felt he was well on his way to healing in more ways than one.

* * *

Caleb had lost count of how many days had passed since Rebecca got ill.

His wheat needed to be harvested, but he couldn't bring himself to leave the house. When he wasn't with Rebecca, he was at Avery's side trying to comfort her.

If Lily and his ma hadn't been there, he couldn't have coped at all.

He stared out the window, torn in two.

"Caleb?" Lily walked up behind him. "I'm here. You gotta do what you have to in order to keep the farm runnin'."

He turned to face her. "How'd you know that was in my head?"

"Cuz I'd be thinkin' the same thing if I was in charge a the crops. That wheat won't be any good if you don't harvest it soon. Is there anyone you can hire to help?"

"When Mr. Iverson came by to check on us, he said there's a man stayin' at the hotel lookin' for work. I reckon I could get him."

"Then, do it."

"But—"

"But nothin'. Your ma an' me can tend Rebecca an' Avery. Lucas is fine now. In another day or two, he might be able to help you outside."

Caleb found himself staring at her, so he quickly shifted his eyes. Her strength had impressed him from the start, but she'd grown into an even more incredible woman.

"I know you're right." He moved a little closer to her. "But you hafta swear that if I'm out workin' an' there's any change at all, you'll come get me."

"Course I will."

"All right, then." He glanced down the quiet hallway. Seemed everyone was asleep. "I'll go now. Hopefully that man at Iverson's will still be there."

She smiled and lit up the room.

He raced out the door before his thoughts took him elsewhere.

* * *

"Lily." Rebecca tried to push her voice as loud as she could, but it didn't come out well.

She tried again. "Lily." Since speaking hadn't worked, she let out a groan with much more volume.

Lily raced into the room. "You sound awful. What hurts?"

Rebecca patted the bed. "Sit."

"Oh, sweetie. You shouldn't even try to talk, but I'll get close so I can hear you." She climbed onto the bed and sat on a pillow right beside Rebecca's head.

"Thank you."

"It's fine. This pillow is comfortable."

"Not what I meant." Rebecca took several slow breaths. "Thank you for bein' here."

It was unreal that she'd said those words, but she'd grown to love Lily. If things had been different, it would've been nice to have her as a best friend. Under the circumstances, Lily would have to become more than that.

"I told you I'd stay if you got sick." Lily smiled and pushed a strand of hair from Rebecca's face. "But don't get too used to me. I gotta go home sometime."

Rebecca touched a hand to her chest. "It's gettin' harder to breathe. The air feels heavy."

Lily's smile vanished. "I best be cookin' more onions."

"Not yet." She turned her head on the pillow to look at her friend. "I'm worn out, Lily. I know I'm dyin'."

"Hush. Don't say that."

"I need to." Rebecca took a deep breath through her nose, then blew it out her mouth. This wasn't easy to say. "I want you to take care a my family. I know you love Caleb." Another breath. "Can you love my little girl?"

Tears streamed down Lily's cheeks. "Please don't talk like that. You can't give up. That's part a healin', you gotta try with all your might." She sucked in staggered breaths and grasped Rebecca's hand. "Stop talkin' 'bout dyin'."

"It's important. If I know they'll be with someone good, I can pass in peace."

"I said, stop." Lily grabbed onto her and held her. "You feel like my sister. Part a my family. An' I don't wanna lose you."

"Lily."

Lily let her go and sat upright, wiping her eyes. "This ain't right."

"Maybe it's how it was always supposed to be. If this hadn't happened, you an' Caleb may never a seen each other again. You need each other."

"He's *your* husband."

"But he loves *you*. I want him to be happy." Rebecca rubbed her aching chest. "Soon, I'll be with Abraham again."

"No. Stop sayin' things like that."

Rebecca reached for Lily's hand. "You're a believer, aren't you?"

"Yes."

"Then you know sumthin' better is waitin' for me. I'm not afraid to die, I just hate the pain."

Lily stroked the top of her hand. "I'll see if Doc Garrison can get you sumthin' for that. I don't want you to hurt."

"Thank you. But remember what I said. An' when the time comes an' Avery is old enough to understand . . . tell her 'bout me."

Lily hugged her again—not so hard this time—then got off the bed. "I'm gonna make you a poultice, then I'll see if Mrs. Henry can go to Doc Garrison for that medicine. If he's decent, maybe he'll come here an' look in on you."

Rebecca nodded, then shut her eyes. Sleep was the only way she escaped her misery.

The other night, she'd had a dream. Perhaps a *vision*. Abraham had come to her and beckoned her home. She'd tried to reach for his hand, but couldn't quite grasp it. And when she woke, she remembered him telling her . . .

Soon.

Chapter 32

Caleb wrapped an arm over Lucas's shoulder. "I ain't never seen anyone manage a scythe the way you do. You did great."

"Yeah? Thanks." Lucas smiled. His smirk hadn't been seen in a great while.

This was the boy Caleb remembered, who was quickly becoming a man.

They headed inside to share the good news with the rest of the family. They still had threshing to do, but at least the wheat was cut.

His ma opened the back door for them. Her dismal expression changed everything.

Caleb grabbed her arm. "Has sumthin' happened? Why didn't you come an' fetch us?"

She held up her hands. "There wasn't time. Doc Garrison just left. He told me what we can expect."

"Is Lily with Becca?"

"Yes. An' the children are in Avery's room. I looked in on 'em a few moments ago, an' they're fine. Doc said we was blessed that Avery's case was mild."

Caleb rubbed his temples. "What else did he say?"

"Let's sit." She took a chair, and Caleb dropped into his own.

Rebecca hadn't shown any improvement for days. Lily's poultices hadn't worked as they had for Lucas. She'd told him that she thought Rebecca didn't have the strength to cough out the phlegm. Nothing helped.

His ma swallowed hard. "She's dyin', Caleb." She sniffled and silent tears dripped onto the table.

He covered his face with his hands and rocked back and forth. Lucas placed a hand on his back, but said nothing.

Every breath Caleb took came out harder and faster. He couldn't think. Everything became a blur.

His ma lightly tapped the table in front of him. "Doc Garrison gave her some morphine to ease the pain. If you want to speak to her, you'd best do it now. Soon, she won't be aware."

Her words sunk deep. He rapidly nodded and got up from the chair.

His ma grabbed his hand and cradled it to her face. "I know, son. This is the hardest thing you'll ever do."

He kissed her cheek, then rushed to Rebecca.

The room they'd shared for nearly two years seemed foreign. It had become a death chamber, and he hated it.

Lily sat in a chair on the opposite side of the bed. Her face was red and swollen. When she saw him, she dropped her head, looking completely defeated. He could tell she'd been crying for some time and hadn't stopped.

"I'm sorry, Caleb." Her voice shook. "I tried."

A single nod was all he could manage. He turned all his attention to his wife and knelt on the bed beside her.

Lily stood and ran her hand along Rebecca's arm, then walked away, sobbing.

For a brief second, he nearly called her back, feeling the need for her strength and support. But as Lily had shown by leaving, he should spend these precious moments alone with Rebecca.

"Becca?" He laid down and clung to her. "Can you hear me?"

"Caleb." She rasped his name. "Abraham . . . is waitin'."

"No. I don't want you to go." He sobbed and clutched on tighter as if that alone could keep her there.

"It's my time." She lifted a trembling hand to his face. "Let me go."

"I failed you." His chest ached so much he swore it had ripped apart. "I coulda done a whole lot better."

"You did your best." Every word she breathed out grew more and more faint. "That's all anyone can do."

His best. There had to be more he could've done. More words spoken in love. More time spent together.

He stroked her face—still beautiful regardless of the lesions. "What'll I do now?"

Her eyes had nearly shut, her breathing slowed to the point of almost being absent. "Take Avery."

He sucked in air, wishing with all his heart that he could pass it on to her, then he kissed her dry cracked lips.

Somehow, she managed to lift the corners of her mouth into a smile. "Caleb."

He leaned close and closed his eyes.

Her lips touched his ear. "Be with . . . Lily . . ." Her body went limp.

"Becca . . . ?" Caleb sobbed until darkness set in.

* * *

Though exhausted, Lily couldn't sleep. She'd cried till her eyes had almost swollen shut. Hearing Caleb's mournful sobs made her tears fall faster. She shared his pain.

Mrs. Henry was no better. She'd been trying to remain calm for the sake of the children, but even they'd done their fair share of mourning. They were so young that Lily believed they whimpered not so much from the understanding of what had happened, but because everyone they loved was hurting.

At least they'd fallen asleep.

Lily tossed aside her blanket and crept to the children's bedroom. Avery and Noah were cuddled next to each other. Mrs. Henry lay facing the wall on the opposite side of Avery. Lily assumed she was still awake but too numb to move.

Lily was tempted to pick Noah up, but she left him there. He looked content and at peace.

She assumed Lucas was in his room, but hadn't seen him all night. Caleb had told her he'd been doing well working the fields. Right now, her brother was the least of her worries.

When Rebecca passed, it had been too late to go for the mortician. Caleb had covered her lifeless body with a blanket, shut the bedroom door, and had been sitting in the hallway leaning against it ever since.

Lily tiptoed down the hallway and sat beside him.

They said nothing. Just stared into the darkness and waited for morning.

* * *

Lily startled and popped her eyes open. Her head rested on Caleb's shoulder. It took her a moment to recall where they were.

She stood and everything came painfully back to her. "Caleb?"

When he lifted his head, she witnessed a shattered man. He didn't say a word, only looked at her through swollen lids.

"We need to get the mortician."

He pushed himself up from the floor and trudged to the kitchen.

She followed him. "Caleb? Did you hear me?"

"I gotta check the wheat."

She grabbed both of his arms and stared into his face. "Forget the wheat. It's done. You gotta fetch someone to come an' take Rebecca."

His eyes misted over. "Is she really gone?"

"Yes. I'm sorry, Caleb."

He grabbed onto her so tight, it took her breath. "Becca was so good. She didn't deserve to die like this." He cried and held on, grasping Lily as if holding onto everything he'd ever lost.

"I know. But she was hurtin', an' now the pain is gone."

Caleb let her go and stepped back. "Not for me, Lily." He held his head with both hands. "My mind ain't workin' right."

Lucas walked in, but turned to leave the instant he saw them.

"Lucas." Lily motioned him back. "I was gettin' worried 'bout you. I'm glad to see you."

"Why?" He firmed his jaw, looking as miserable as Caleb. "This is all my fault. You said I could start over, but no matter what I do, I hurt folks. If I hadn't come here, Rebecca would still be alive."

Caleb's head tipped to one side and he moved closer to Lucas.

Lucas's eyes widened and he took a step back, but then he stood tall and squared his shoulders. "Go on, you can hit me. Kill me if you hafta for makin' your wife sick. I deserve it."

"I ain't gonna hit you or come anywhere close to killin' you."

Lily breathed easier, but the tension in the room hadn't lessened.

Caleb put one hand on Lucas's shoulder. "Bringin' my sick son here, changed all our lives in ways we coulda never imagined. Some good an' some bad. But don't think you made Rebecca die. Doc Garrison said there was other things wrong with her. She likely wouldn't a lived more than another year. The pox just sped up the process."

Lucas's brows drew tight. "You mean, she was dyin' anyways?"

"That's right." Caleb took a huge breath. "If you would, I'd like you to go with me to the mortician. I could use you by my side."

Lucas bobbed his head. Every trace of fear and regret melted away from his features.

Caleb turned to Lily. "Kiss the kids for me, an' let 'em know I'll see 'em soon."

Lily choked down more tears. "I will."

The two men walked out side by side. A sight Lily would never forget.

* * *

Nearly a month had passed since Lily had arrived in Waynesville.

They'd buried Rebecca next to Abraham, the Henry boy Lily hadn't met, but who'd made an impact on many lives.

Rebecca passed away not knowing the truth about how Abraham had died, but Lily had told Caleb she thought it was best. Some things didn't need to be said.

And even though Rebecca had wanted Lily to be with Caleb and Avery, it didn't seem right. Lily had to go home to the cove, and their home was in Waynesville. Besides, she was certain Mrs. Henry would stay with Caleb and the child. They'd get plenty of loving care.

Lucas had gone into town to hire a driver, and Lily wandered the property with Noah in her arms, getting her thoughts together.

"Wanna swing?" She headed that direction.

"Swing." Noah pointed and grinned.

They'd been on it before. Of course, the first time Noah had experienced it, he'd been on his pa's lap.

Guilt weighed heavy on Lily, but what other choice did she have but to leave?

She let the May sunshine warm them and enjoyed the breeze created by their motion.

"I'll get your grampa to help me fix up one a these when we get home." She pumped her legs a little harder. "I bet you'll be glad to see Isaac an' Horace again. I know I will." She kept a firm hold on her son. "Oh, an' your auntie Violet of course."

"Sissy."

"No, *auntie*. Can you say that? Auntie."

"Attee."

"Close enough."

Mrs. Henry approached with Avery by the hand.

"Avee," Noah said. "Sissy."

"Oh, my goodness, son. Things are much too confusin'."

Avery jerked away from her gramma and ran to the swing. "Mine."

Noah giggled, but then fussed when Lily set him on the ground. "It's Avery's turn." Avery crawled into her lap and clung on.

Noah rushed over to his gramma. The child didn't lack attention.

"I'm gonna miss you," Lily whispered in Avery's ear. The sweet girl had been spending a lot of time in Lily's arms since Rebecca had died.

"Where's Caleb?" his ma asked.

"I reckon he's walkin' the fields." Lily stopped the swing. "He's strugglin' with the idea of Noah leavin'."

"He ain't the only one." Mrs. Henry frowned. "An' you know very well that it ain't only Noah he's gonna miss."

Lily got up from the swing with Avery glued to her. "We've talked 'bout this." She covered the girl's ears. "He's still mournin' Rebecca. I'm only complicatin' things."

"She wanted the two a you together. She told me herself."

"She told me, too, but it ain't right. Least not now. Maybe in time . . ."

"Time." The woman huffed. "Rebecca was proof that we never know how much we'll have. Why waste it?"

Lily knew a little something about mourning. "Caleb's greatest problem has always been guilt. He told me that he let you know 'bout Abraham an' how he died. Caleb shared that sad story with me when he came to the cove. It tore him up, an' he felt worthless and guilty. Then he felt guilty for marryin' Rebecca an' for leavin' me high an' dry. He doesn't need any more guilt."

"But what's that got to do with grievin' Rebecca?"

"If I stayed with Caleb now, it wouldn't take long 'fore he started mopin'. Feelin' guilty. He'd tell himself he jumped into sumthin' without givin' himself time to let go a her. I ain't gonna do that to him."

Mrs. Henry stroked Noah's back. "You know my son better than he knows himself." Again, she huffed. "Fine. Go on an' leave. But mark my words, you ain't seen the last of us." She placed a hand on Avery's head. "All *three* of us."

A team of horses pulling a wagon approached. Lucas's red hair shimmered in the sunlight. He sat next to a scruffy-looking driver.

"Do you know that man?" Lily pointed.

"Yes. That's old Mr. Kershaw. He looks bad, but he's decent." She frowned and crossed her arms. "He'll get you home just fine."

They pulled to a stop not far from Lily.

Lucas hopped down. "Ready to go?"

"Yep. I'm all packed. What little I had. But I need to find Caleb, so he can tell Noah goodbye."

"Lucas." Mrs. Henry said. "Why don't you come inside with me? I can pack up some food for y'all to take. An' Lily. We hafta switch babies."

Avery shook her head. "No."

"Sweetie," Lily said. "I gotta go. Now go to your gramma."

Lucas took Noah from Mrs. Henry, then she pried Avery away from Lily. The child had been holding on so tight, it felt like Lily was shedding a second skin.

Avery fussed, but Lily knew in time she'd be fine.

Lucas put Noah in Lily's arms. "I already told Caleb goodbye. I reckon I'll see him again someday." He grinned and followed Mrs. Henry into the house.

Lily gave a quick wave to the driver, then headed to the field.

With every step, her heart grew heavier. Why did doing the right thing have to hurt so bad?

She found Caleb in the middle of the cut fields, simply staring toward the sky.

His broad shoulders drooped low.

Lily took a breath and built up her courage. "I've come to say goodbye. Noah, too."

Caleb didn't move an inch. "I don't want to."

"But Lucas just got back with the driver, an' we gotta go."

Caleb's shoulders lifted and fell several times as if he'd taken extremely large breaths. Ever-so-slowly, he spun to face her. Dirty tears smudged his face. "I thought I was done cryin', but I was wrong."

Seeing him this way certainly didn't help ease her into leaving. Her own tears bubbled up and spilled over. "Me, too."

He took a step closer. "I ain't gonna tell you goodbye."

"But—"

"I ain't."

Noah reached out to him, and Caleb took him and cuddled him close. "I love this boy." Caleb pinched his eyes shut and pushed out a stream of droplets. When his lids reopened, he looked at her so intensely it touched her soul. "You know I love you, Lily."

"Caleb. Don't say it." Her tears streamed.

"Do you know what Rebecca's last word was?"

She shook her head.

"It was *Lily*. She told me to be with you." He put his hand to Lily's face. "I know she wanted you to raise Avery. Bring these two up like brother an' sister."

"She told me that very thing. But . . . I can't stay."

His features tightened. "Don't you love me anymore?"

"You know I do. I never stopped. But you need time, an' I'm gonna give it to you." She swallowed hard and took Noah from him. "Tell your pa goodbye."

"Pa." Again, Noah reached for him.

Caleb kissed his cheek, but didn't take him. "I ain't gonna say it." He stood firm.

"You know where we'll be." Lily held onto her son and ran as fast as she could.

She didn't look back.

Chapter 33

Mr. Kershaw was indeed decent. And quite the story-teller. He made the trip a lot more enjoyable for Lucas. In fact, Lily believed this was the happiest she'd ever seen her brother. He sat tall in the seat and genuinely smiled.

It made sense. His burdens had been lifted by true forgiveness.

At least her two companions kept her mind on other things. If she thought about Caleb and the look in his eyes when she'd left, it was too painful.

Of course, Noah occupied a great deal of her time. He'd gotten to where he no longer cowered around Lucas, and Lucas took extra care in his actions toward the child.

As they neared the cove, things got a bit quieter.

Lucas pointed at the Quincy's house. "Old Mr. Quincy was shot near the end a the war. His grandsons used to blow a horn to let us know when the soldiers was comin'. I'd always hear it first, then let my family know."

"That's right," Lily said. "Then Lucas would tuck a hen under each arm, an' I'd take the pig. We had to hide the livestock, so the soldiers wouldn't take 'em."

Mr. Kershaw rubbed his gray beard. "I was too old to fight in the war, but I seen a lot a bad things in my day." He gazed around him. "Best to put all the ugly things behind us. This is a fine place. You're lucky to have a home here."

"Yep, we are." Lily breathed in the fresh air. "What do you think, Noah? Are you happy to be home?"

"Home." He leaned backward and giggled. "Home." He stretched out his arms and wiggled his fingers.

The cabin must've looked funny upside down.

Mr. Kershaw steered the team close to the barn. Lily cupped a hand over her eyes and peered at the distant creek. Beyond it, a new grave marker stuck up above a large mound of rock-covered dirt.

Lucas touched her arm. "Reckon that's Ma?"

"Yep." She smoothed a hand over his head. "We'll go later. Let's go see Pa an' the boys."

They stepped to the ground and Mr. Kershaw handed them their belongings. "I'm gonna get goin' myself, while I still got lots a daylight."

"Thank you." Lily gave him a quick hug, then eyed him closely. "Have you got enough food to get you back home?"

"Plenty. I always come prepared."

Lily smiled and nodded. "Please let the Henrys know we made it home safe."

"I will." He patted Lucas on the back. "Take care, son."

"You, too. An' try to avoid all them ruts goin' back." Lucas winked.

Mr. Kershaw grunted and returned to his wagon. His chuckles carried through the air.

Lily put her arm around her brother and they headed for the cabin.

"You know," she said. "The boys ain't gonna know what to think a you. Go easy on 'em, all right?"

"I will. I'll try to be the brother they shoulda had all along. Maybe act more like Caleb."

"Pa," Noah said.

Lily assumed he'd reacted to Lucas's remark, but then looked up and saw her pa approaching.

"Pa!" Noah cried out louder this time and reached for the man. It would take a bit of work, but she intended to set everyone in the family straight as to who was who.

Her pa latched onto him with his ever-so-strong arm and hugged him tight. "Look at you! You've grown at least six inches."

Lily rolled her eyes. "Hey, Pa."

With Noah still in the crook of his arm, he moved toward her.

She hugged him, then nodded toward Lucas. "He's promised to help work the farm. He helped Caleb cut the wheat in Waynesville. Did a good job, too."

Lucas lowered his head and inched forward. "I know what I done was wrong, Pa. I aim to make up for it."

The man nodded and gestured to the house. "Isaac an' Horace have been countin' the days."

Excitement flooded through Lily, and she flung the door open. She gasped and her eyes popped wide. "Violet?"

Her sister burst into tears and almost bowled Lily over. "Lily!"

Within seconds, Lily was surrounded with hugs and kisses. Her pa stood back laughing.

Lily stared at her beautiful sister. "How'd you know to be here?"

"Gideon's been watchin' for you. He spotted the wagon in the valley, then hightailed it to fetch me. He an' Stardust have become best friends."

Gideon sauntered over, leaning on his crutch. "Surprise."

Lily placed a hand to Violet's belly. "Look at you. How much longer?"

"Two more months. Plenty a time to make things for the baby. Will you help me?"

Lily hugged her again. "There's nothin' else I'd rather do."

"Wanna play charades?" Horace asked and strutted like a rooster.

Lily laughed. "Not right now, maybe later." Overwhelmed didn't describe her feelings well enough.

There was only one dark spot in the small cabin. Lucas hung back in the corner. Lily hated that he felt so out of place. But all things took time, and he had amends to make. Especially with his little brothers.

Lily motioned to the kitchen table. "Let's all sit down an' talk. There's things that need to be said."

Her pa's brows crinkled, but he complied.

Everyone sat, and Lily held Noah on her lap. He grinned and patted the tabletop.

Lily gazed around the table at all the smiling faces. She belonged here. "When I came home an' found Ma sick an' Noah gone, I thought I'd never be happy again."

Noah turned his head and looked up at her. "Ma."

Violet's hand shot to her mouth, Horace's eyes opened wide, and their pa shook his head.

Isaac's nose wrinkled. "Why'd he call you Ma?"

"Cuz I am his ma."

"Huh?"

Lily looked to her pa and he nodded for her to continue. "See . . . when I found out I was gonna have a baby, Ma an' Pa knew I wasn't ready to be a ma. I wasn't married an' . . . well. It just wasn't my time. So they decided to tell folks that Noah was their little boy an' my brother. They thought it would be less confusin'."

"So . . ." Isaac looked upward, then nudged Horace. "Noah ain't our brother."

"That's right, but he's part a our family. He's your nephew."

"Can he still play with us?"

"Course he can." Lily smiled at her sweet brother.

"Is he gonna live here?" Horace asked.

"We all will, long as Pa don't care. Do you Pa?"

"Yeah," Lucas said. "Do you Pa?"

"Course not. This is your home. I want you here. All of you." He directed the last remark at Lucas.

Finally, he sat a little taller. Just as he had in the wagon.

"That also means," her pa said, "that Noah needs to call me Grampa. It's high time."

Isaac got up from his chair and leaned over to Noah's level. "Can you say Grampa?"

"Gappa."

Her pa laughed. "I can be Gappa. I kinda like it."

"Gappa." Noah giggled.

Lily's heart rested. The boys had accepted the situation easier than she'd expected. Because of their youth, they likely didn't grasp the concept of an unmarried pregnant woman. They hadn't even asked who Noah's pa was. It appeared that they were simply happy that everyone was together again.

The conversation shifted to many other things. Lily told tales of her time in St. Louis and happier stories about living with the Jacobsons in Asheville.

Violet and Gideon shared details of their wedding and ideas they had for baby names, and eventually they all shared thoughts about their ma.

Lily wasn't ready to talk about Caleb just yet. She intended to wait till she could be alone with Violet. That particular story was private, meant only to be shared with her sister and dearest friend.

* * *

Violet and Gideon had returned home, and Lily settled into her old room, along with Noah. The boys argued that he should be in the loft, but since Lucas was back, he took that particular bed, much to the grumblings of Isaac and Horace.

She assured Lucas that in time the boys wouldn't fear him, but he needed to find a way to regain their trust. Lucas promised them a bed-time story, which they found strange, but not terrorizing them was a step in the right direction.

Lily tucked Noah into bed, kissed him goodnight, then crept from the room. She kept the door slightly ajar.

Her pa was sitting in his old rocker in front of the fireplace. Had it not been for the addition of Noah and the absence of her ma, things would feel completely the same as they'd been long ago.

She tucked her legs beneath her and sat on the sofa. "You doin' all right?"

"Fit as a frog."

She chuckled. "Truly, Pa? How are you gettin' by?"

"I miss Rose, but I know she's happier now." He turned his head and smiled. "Now that you an' our boy is back, things will perk up 'round here." He cleared his throat. "How are you farin'? You ain't said nothin' 'bout Caleb. Was he kind to you?"

"Yes, Pa. An' his wife was sumthin' special."

"Gideon said the same. Such a shame what happened to her. Lucas should be ashamed a hisself for what he done."

Lily reached for his hand. "Pa? I promise, Lucas has changed. He's tryin' real hard. Caleb told him that Rebecca had other things wrong with her. She woulda died even if Lucas hadn't brought the pox."

He patted her hand and sighed. "I hope you're right 'bout that boy. I told Violet once that I was hard on him so he'd learn. Seems to me, the lesson he got outta all this hit him harder than a brick." He gazed toward the ceiling, then turned and smiled. "If Caleb can forgive him, then I reckon I should, too."

"That's good, Pa."

"An' since we're speakin' a Caleb, you should know that Gideon hasn't stopped talkin' 'bout him. I reckon Violet's gettin' tired a hearin' it."

Lily didn't want to talk about him anymore. She took the opportunity to change the subject. "Are Gideon an' Violet happy?"

"Happy as larks. She fusses at him, but in a good way. They're well-suited." He rocked a bit faster. "So, when should I expect Caleb to arrive?"

"Pa!" She blurted it out without thinking, then covered her mouth, fearing she'd rouse Noah. Why'd their conversation have to go back to Caleb? "What makes you say that?" she whispered.

"Well, it makes sense, don't it? He ain't got a wife no more, an' you ain't got no husband. You have two children that need a ma *and* a pa. 'Sides that, you still love him." He pointed a stiff finger. "An' don't try an' tell me you don't."

She squirmed in the seat, then sat up tall. "Let me ask you sumthin'. It ain't been long since Ma died. How long would you hafta grieve 'fore you'd be ready to move on with someone new?"

"I ain't gonna do that. 'Sides, them's two different situations. Caleb already has a relationship with you. I don't know no women I care to marry."

"But if one came along, could you love someone else?"

He waved his hand. "Ain't gonna happen. I'm too old an' ornery for anyone but your ma. She's gone. End a story."

Lily scooted down and lay comfortably on the sofa. She listened to the creak of the rocker, her pa's steady breathing, and giggles coming from overhead.

Lucas seemed to have won his brothers over with an entertaining story.

Lily shut her eyes, content to be home.

* * *

Violet paced back and forth in the tiny weaner house. Three steps one direction, then three steps back again.

"Come to bed, Violet." Gideon patted the spot beside him. "You need your rest."

"I can't get Lily off my mind. Now that the boys know 'bout Noah, it'll spread all over the cove. Mrs. Quincy will have a heyday with the news." She worked her lower lip with her teeth. "We gotta get Caleb here. That's all there is to it. So he can make an honest woman outta Lily."

"More than a year an' a half after the fact?"

Violet kneeled on the edge of the bed. "That don't matter. They should be together. From what you told me, Caleb still loves her. An' she's loved him regardless of bein' hurt. I hate his wife died an' all, but . . ."

"Lily was right to leave him." Gideon jerked his head back. "Don't glare at me like that. What I meant was, she was right 'bout him needin' time to grieve."

Violet climbed underneath the covers and nestled into her husband. She'd hated being alone in the bed when he was gone. "What did you think of Caleb's ma? She's a widow, ain't she?"

He gave her a sideways glance. "She is. Been one for a number a years. But I can tell you're schemin'. What's on your mind, Violet?"

"She's a widow. Pa is, too."

"He's a widower. Not a widow."

Violet ran her fingers across Gideon's chest. "You knew what I meant."

"You shouldn't be thinkin' that. Like Caleb, your pa just lost his wife. The wounds are too fresh."

She placed a few tiny kisses on his shoulder. "Is Mrs. Henry pretty?"

"Violet." He frowned and shook his head, then relaxed against his pillow. His eyes cut in her direction and he thrummed his fingers on top of the blankets. "All right, I'll tell you. She's comely for her age. Gray-haired, but she keeps it nice. An' I probably shouldn't say it, but she's finer-lookin' than your ma was. Regardless, how can you be thinkin' of someone replacin' your ma so soon?"

"I ain't tryin' to disrespect her memory or Rebecca's neither. I just don't like to think a anyone alone, that's all."

"Hey!" Gideon scooted over. "Did you just poke me in the ribs?"

She giggled. "That was the baby, silly." She grabbed his hand and placed it on her stomach. "Feel that?"

"That's amazin'." He slowly glided his hand all around her belly. "It's flippin' an' floppin'."

"Yep." She cuddled down again. "Can't wait till it's born." The best thought ever struck her and she sat bolt upright. "My wish is comin' true."

"Which one?"

"Lily's home. We can raise our children together. One great big family." Sighing, she lay back.

She meant what she'd said about not wanting to disrespect the dead, but life was too short for anyone to be alone. Even so, out of respect, she'd wait a few weeks, then write a letter and pour her heart out. Hopefully, she could be persuasive.

Chapter 34

Caleb stretched out on the sofa and hoisted one leg over the back. He couldn't get comfortable, but he wasn't about to sleep in the bed he'd shared with Rebecca. He hadn't even gone in the room since the day the mortician had taken her away. The door had remained shut and locked.

He considered the guestroom, but even that part of the house held bad memories. If he wanted to be honest with himself, he chose the sofa because Lily had slept there.

His ma crept in and stood beside him. "I finally got Avery to sleep. That poor baby doesn't know what to think."

"It's been a month. I thought she'd do better by now."

"A month ain't long enough when her life has been turned on its head. She needs a ma."

Caleb sat up and put his head in his hands. "I know."

"An' you also know the solution."

He looked up to find his ma with her arms crossed, staring at him. A stance he knew well. "Ma, you of all people shouldn't be pushin' me like this. You loved Rebecca as much as I did. Probably more."

She sat down and put an arm around his waist. "Yes. An' though I didn't see things clearly at the time, I know now I never shoulda pushed you into marryin' her. You told me you loved

Lily. I couldn't imagine any woman finer than Rebecca. I assumed you was just bein' a silly lovesick boy who didn't know no better. I was wrong."

He tipped his head to look in her eyes. "Maybe so, but I still made the choice to marry her. We can't change any a that now."

"But don't you see?" She cupped a hand to his cheek. "God's givin' you an' Lily another chance. Search your heart. Don't you wanna be with her? Noah, too?"

"I don't hafta do no searchin'. Course I wanna be with them. But we live here. They live there. It's impossible."

His ma threw up her hands. "I swanee, son! Can't you see the bigger picture? Do you love this farm more than you love Lily?"

"That's a silly question."

"Then what's keepin' you here? Are you worried folks might talk? Do you fear they'd think less a you if you took another bride?"

He stared at his lap. "I hate leavin' Becca."

"Caleb." His ma grasped onto his hands, covering them with her own. "She ain't here no more. I can almost guarantee that she an' Abraham are lookin' down on us right now. They'd want the best for their daughter, an' that's Lily. Rebecca gave both of you her blessin's 'fore she died. You ain't got nothin' to feel guilty 'bout no more."

She stood. "T'morra mornin', go to the cemetery. Talk to Rebecca an' your brother. I know it might sound foolish, but I promise, it'll help." She headed toward the hallway. "Goodnight, Caleb. I love you, son."

Before he could respond, she went into Avery's room and shut the door. She hadn't moved back into the guestroom, stating that Avery needed her. But obviously a gramma alone wasn't enough for his daughter.

* * *

It seemed fitting for a light rain to be falling as Caleb walked through town to the cemetery. Not only did it reflect his mood, it reminded him of the time he'd come searching for Rebecca to tell her he was ready to start over.

Something he was about to tell her again.

He'd been up most of the night, working things out in his mind.

Mr. Poe—the man who'd helped him harvest the wheat—had expressed interest in purchasing a farm of his own. From Caleb's understanding, he was still staying at Iverson's. Caleb intended to stop there on his way back home.

For many nights after Rebecca died, he'd dreamed about her. Lately, all his dreams had been of Lily.

His ma had told him he had nothing more to feel guilty about, so why did it creep in every time Lily came to mind?

With his head bent low, he followed the path through the cemetery to where his wife and brother had been laid to rest.

Caleb's heart wrenched, and he dropped to his knees.

Freshly cut lilies rested atop Rebecca's grave.

"Where'd they come from?" He glanced around, but no one was in sight. His ma was at home with Avery, so she couldn't have done it.

He shut his eyes.

"Can I go to her? Is it right for me to leave so soon an' be with Lily?"

With his lids pinched tight, he tipped his head back and let the rain wash over him. A breeze blew and something brushed against his hand on his lap.

One of the lilies lay at his fingertips.

His heart beat hard. Emotion overwhelmed him, but no tears came. He'd been mourning for what felt like forever, and it had become part of him. He'd started grieving long before Rebecca's death. It'd begun the day he'd pulled the trigger on Abraham.

"Be with Lily."

Rebecca's final words came to the forefront of his mind. Yes, she'd given her blessing, and as his ma had reminded him, Rebecca was no longer there. Her body might be lying below him, but her soul lived on elsewhere.

He envisioned her and Abraham walking hand in hand by a sparkling river. His vision also held a swing that hung from a large oak tree, where Abraham could push Rebecca and bring out her never-ending smile.

With the lily clutched in his hand, Caleb moved to his brother's grave. "Love her forever, Abraham."

The rain stopped.

Smiling, Caleb headed for the hotel.

Mrs. Iverson met him with a frown. "You've been to the graves, ain't ya?" She nodded at the lily. "It's beautiful. Them kind are hard to come by this time a year. Where'd you find it?"

"I didn't. There was a bunch of them layin' on Rebecca's grave. I don't know who put them there, but I'm happy they did."

She clutched her bosom. "Bless your heart. I know you miss her."

"I do, but she's in a finer place." He took a deep breath. "Is Mr. Poe still stayin' here?"

"Yep. Room nine. I think he's in. He usually don't go out too early."

"Thank you." He gestured down the hallway. "Reckon it's all right if I check in on him?"

"I doubt he's sleepin', so go on an' knock. You got more work to be done?"

"You could say that." He cast a broad smile, only to receive an odd look from Mrs. Iverson.

Maybe it wasn't right to wear even a slightly happy expression so soon after losing his wife, but it felt appropriate.

"Oh. Caleb?" Mrs. Iverson lifted some papers and pulled out an envelope. "This came for you. I was gonna come by later and deliver it, but since you're here, you'll save me the trip."

He took it from her.

She stepped back and folded her arms. "Looks like them folks in Cades Cove wanna stay in touch. I believe that writin's a woman's." Her eyes formed into slits. "Be sure to tell your ma I said hey."

"I will." He tucked the letter into his pocket. It had to be from Lily. He ached to read it, but he needed to see Mr. Poe first.

He headed down the hallway and knocked on the door.

* * *

Caleb walked away from Iverson's feeling lighter than air. Truthfully, he was a bit surprised that he'd been able to give up what he'd put so much work into, but Mr. Poe had made a fair offer and Caleb had followed his heart and readily accepted it.

Lily might not expect him so soon, but her final words were a sure sign she thought he'd be there eventually. Just the idea of seeing her again set his heart racing.

He'd been so thrilled that his meeting with Mr. Poe went well that he'd nearly forgotten the letter. He pulled it from his pocket and opened it.

The penmanship was impressive, but it wasn't from Lily. It had been written by Violet. Though disappointed, he stopped in the middle of the road to read it. A small amount of fear crept in, worried that something might've happened to Lily—or perhaps Noah.

Mr. Kershaw had let Caleb and his ma know that he'd safely delivered them to the cove. Even so . . .

He quickly read.

Dear Caleb,

I know you did not expect to hear from me, but I felt compelled to write and let you know my feelings.

He stopped reading.

"She hates me," he mumbled, then lifted the letter again.

When you left the cove, Lily told me about her feelings for you. Then when she discovered she was with child, she prayed every day for your return.

I read the letter you sent telling her of your plans to marry someone else. I admit, I hated you then. I could not understand how someone I thought was kind could be so cold-hearted.

Every word cut deep, but he kept on reading.

I also could not comprehend why Lily kept claiming love for you. Not after you had hurt her so badly. She told me there were things I would never understand, but that she would always love you.

Now that I am a married woman, I understand love more so than when I was a silly girl with dreams of the perfect man. Gideon has blessed my life in more ways than I can count. I cannot envision being without him. We have become a part of each other.

Lily's heart has been joined with yours for a very long time. She needs you, and so does Noah. I know you need them, too.

When Gideon and I married, his folks gave us a small cabin to live in and establish ourselves. It suits us for now, but eventually we'll build something larger. With our baby coming, we will require more room.

If you would be willing to live in the cove, I know my pa would give you land and the help you need to build a cabin for you, Lily, and your children. And if you're so inclined to bring her, your ma is more than welcome.

He reread the last line, shook his head, then finished the letter.

Please give my suggestion your consideration. Lily told me what it was like spending the final days with your wife. She said what a lovely person she was and also talked about your sweet daughter.

I don't hate you any longer, Caleb. You are the one person who can make my sister truly happy. I want that for her. Besides, Noah needs his pa.

Folks in the cove have been made aware that Lily is Noah's ma. No one has asked her to reveal who you are, but I know it would make her life easier if you married her. Folks would eventually stop their gossip.

Even with folks talking ugly about her, Lily walks with her head held high. She proudly carries Noah to church and ignores nasty remarks. I don't have to tell you how strong she is.

Lastly, you should know that whatever you did for Lucas has worked wonders. He is the brother I remember from long ago.

Thank you.

With love,

Violet

Caleb placed the letter against his heart and breathed easy. At least she'd said she didn't hate him anymore.

He walked home with renewed energy, knowing he was needed and *wanted* elsewhere.

He found it odd that she'd mentioned his ma, but Violet had always been kind. She probably didn't think his ma should be alone in Waynesville. Of course, Violet didn't know her. His ma was self-sufficient and enjoyed time by herself. Not to mention, she had an abundance of friends.

Still, he'd ask her. She might not care to be so far away from Avery, and he assumed she'd want to stay close to him and Noah, too.

"One big, happy family." Caleb chuckled and rapidly increased his pace.

Chapter 35

Lucas raced into the cabin. "Lily. Mrs. Quincy's comin'." His brows wove up and down. "Sorry." He flew up the stairs.

Lily set aside the tiny baby booties she'd been knitting and stood.

"Want us to go up with Lucas?" Horace asked from the living room.

Isaac peered over the back of the sofa, along with Noah's tiny face.

The sight tickled her, and she giggled. "It's up to you. I can handle Mrs. Quincy just fine."

"But I heard her call Ma a liar," Isaac said. "That ain't nice."

"No it ain't." Lily wandered to the sofa and patted Noah's head. "But words can't hurt us, 'less we let 'em. I don't intend to let that happen."

Noah reached for her. So when Mrs. Quincy knocked on the door, Lily greeted her with him in her arms.

"Well, hello, Mrs. Quincy. It's fine to see you." Lily cast her most pleasant smile.

"Lily." She slightly dipped her head, then eyed Noah like he was a disease. "I came by with a letter for you. It's from Asheville."

She held it out, and Lily nabbed it. "You didn't read it, did you?"

"Heavens no! I would never do such a thing."

"Hmm. I wonder who it's from . . ." She knew full well, but thought she'd probe Mrs. Quincy further.

The woman pointed at the envelope. "Someone named Jacobson."

Lily flipped it over, then back again. "That's odd. I don't see their name on the envelope anywhere. How would you know that?"

"Uh . . ." She scratched the back of her neck. "I admit. I held it up to the light and saw the name through the paper."

"But you didn't open it?"

"*No.* I swear it on the Bible." She firmly nodded, then licked her lips. "I've been curious 'bout sumthin'."

"Yes?"

"Do you have any idea whatever became of that Callie girl?"

Horace snickered.

Lily snapped her head around and glared at him. He clamped a hand over his mouth.

Lily returned her attention to their *guest* and frowned. "The last I heard, Callie died from the pox. Seems it traveled all through the mountains." She jerked her head toward the sofa. "It ain't nothin' to laugh 'bout. Horace was outta line. Weren't you Horace?"

"Yes'm." His acting had somewhat improved. He actually sounded sorry.

Noah reached out and poked Mrs. Quincy in the arm. "Gamma."

Lily patted his leg. "No, honey, she ain't your gramma."

Mrs. Quincy leered down her nose at him. "Who that is remains a mystery, don't it? Course, your dear ma has parted this earth, but I assume there's another gramma somewhere?"

"Waynesville!" Isaac hollered.

Lily shot him a wide-eyed look to hush, so he ducked behind the sofa.

Mrs. Quincy chuckled. "Waynesville, hmm? You're a mystery Lily Larsen."

"Yes, I am. An' I intend to stay that way." She gestured out the door. "Thank you for bringin' the letter."

With her nose stuck high in the air, Mrs. Quincy marched off.

Lily shut the door a bit louder than normal, then whipped around and glared at her brothers. She fisted her hands on her hips. "I shoulda made you boys go upstairs."

"We offered," Horace said.

Isaac poked his head up. "That's right. We offered."

"Well, here." She set Noah on the floor. "You can make up for speakin' outta turn by watchin' Noah for a spell so I can read my letter."

Isaac hopped from the sofa and grabbed his hand. "Let's go to the loft an' see if Lucas has more stories to tell."

The boys sounded like thunder going up the stairs. Fortunately, Isaac took his time with Noah.

She sat at the table and opened the envelope. If Mrs. Quincy had read it, Lily doubted the Jacobsons would say anything that was private, so she wasn't *too* worried.

She read quietly and smiled at every word.

Mr. Jacobson had written it.

Dearest Lily,

We hope this letter finds you well. We miss you terribly, but understand that you are where you need to be. Please write soon and let us know how little Noah is doing. We were sorry to hear about your mother. Hiram shared the sad news. We assume she passed shortly after your arrival.

Lily lowered the letter and rested it on the table. She should've written long ago, but her mind had been on other things. There were many other long-overdue letters as well. She'd make time later.

You will be happy to know that we are attending church regularly again. My sweet Arabelle is singing in the choir. She has always had a lovely voice, and now she's lifting it to the Lord in thanks and praise.

She has also become an exceptional cook. I owe you a great deal of gratitude. However, my waistline is suffering for it.

Lily giggled.

The girls are well. Winnifred still tries to be in charge of the others, but as you know, Genevieve won't allow it. They have their spats, but Arabelle makes certain they hug and make up after every argument.

Opal continues to be our ray of sunshine. Her giggles overcome any sad thoughts that creep into our home. She has also passed on her joyful talent to Levi.

Along with laughter, the boy talks much more now. His mother is working with him and the girls on their letters. Each at their own stage of development. When the children aren't being schooled, they help Arabelle with daily chores. In addition, we both continue to encourage their play time and use of their imaginations.

Know that you are welcome to stay with us any time you wish. We will keep your room clean and ready, even if it is only for a brief visit.

We pray for your health, happiness, and God's blessings,
Arthur Jacobson

Lily held the letter to her heart, beaming. The man most definitely had a way with words. With all the chaos in her life, she hadn't realized how much she missed them. Someday, she'd pay them a visit, but she'd always return to the cove.

* * *

The June weather had proven to be perfect for traveling, but it took a team of four horses to pull Caleb's loaded-down wagon. His ma had insisted on bringing half their furniture.

Honestly, Caleb could've parted with it much easier than he'd let go of his livestock. Aside from the four horses, Mr. Poe bought every animal Caleb owned as well as the farm.

His ma slapped him on the leg. "Why are you frownin'? Ain't we nearly there?"

"I was just thinkin' 'bout them cows."

Avery handed him Moo Cow. "Baby cow." She sat securely between his ma and him and had hardly fussed at all the entire way.

"There you go," his ma said. "You got your cow." She let out a laugh. "Caleb. Stop mopin'. If anyone should be glum, it should be me. I left all my friends behind. The good hotel food. Maids to clean up after me." She sighed. "Now I'm goin' someplace I ain't never been before. What if I don't like it?"

"Then I'll take you back to Waynesville. I'm sure Mr. Iverson would be happy to give you your old room."

She cocked her head, then sat tall. "I s'pose I *could* go back. But maybe I'll decide I like this place. All I've seen is mountains. I thought you said there was some kind a valley."

"There is. Be patient an' you'll see."

When they reached the familiar road leading to the cove, Caleb's insides tumbled. No doubt, nervous excitement.

"Close your eyes, Ma," he said. "You, too, Avery."

His ma reluctantly did his bidding. Avery giggled and copied her.

The landscape opened up, and the lush valley spread out before them. The high mountains framed everything with a border in multiple shades of green.

"Okay. You can open them again." Caleb took Avery's hands away from her eyes.

"Look, Gamma!"

His ma gasped. "Oh, my. I had no idea sumthin' like this could be in the middle a the mountains." She hugged Avery to her. "Baby girl, I think we're gonna like it here."

"Ma?" Caleb gulped. "What do I say to Lily when I see her?"

"You'll know when the time comes."

He prayed she was right.

He guided the horses to the cabin—the place he'd left his heart—and pulled them to a stop.

Laughter came from the nearby creek.

"Get the frog, Noah!"

It sounded like Isaac, but his voice had changed some.

Noah's giggles definitely hadn't.

Avery squirmed and tried to wriggle off the seat. "Noah!"

"I take it your son is playin' with Lily's brothers." His ma stepped to the ground, then reached for Avery. "I think I see Lucas over yonder, too. C'mon, Avery. Let's go see *your* brother." She looked up at Caleb. "I reckon you'll find Lily inside the cabin. It's nearly suppertime. She's likely cookin'."

He bobbed his head, but remained frozen to the seat.

"Go on, Caleb. You've waited a long time for this." She smiled, clutched onto Avery, and walked away.

Caleb eased out of the wagon on shaky legs.

He took slow steps toward the cabin, fearing his feet might fail him. It felt like he'd come home, but until he knew Lily wanted him there, he couldn't calm down.

He rapped several times, then took a step back.

"Mrs. Quincy!" Lily yelled. "If that's you again, you might as well just turn 'round an' go back home!"

Caleb couldn't help but smirk. Violet was right. Lily was as strong as ever.

She swung the door wide, then stumbled backward and landed on her rump.

"Lily!" Caleb dove for her, tripped, and ended up beside her on the floor.

"Caleb?" She stared at him, then grabbed the sides of his face and peered even deeper into his eyes. "You're really here?"

Tears he thought wouldn't come again, fooled him and pooled, clouding his vision. "Yes. Forever if you want me."

"It's all I ever wanted." She wrapped her arms around him and kissed him before he could take a breath. "I love you!"

"I love you, Lily."

Their bodies entwined, and he kissed all over her face, then returned to her perfect lips.

"What in tarnation?"

They both gasped, then gazed upward. Her pa stood over them, loudly tapping his foot.

"Hey, Mr. Larsen." Caleb kept his hold on Lily. "Nice to see you again."

"Why are you an' Lily tumblin' 'round on the floor that way? I seen them kids comin' in from the creek. If they'd a found you like this . . ."

"Sorry, Pa." Lily sat up. "Caleb just got here."

"I can see that. I passed his wagon comin' in from the fields." He shook his head and grinned at Caleb. "You bring all a North Carolina with you?"

"No, sir." Caleb slowly rose to his feet, while keeping hold of Lily's hand. "Just part. I'm here to marry Lily. If she'll have me."

She burrowed against him. "You sure you're ready?"

"He's ready," her pa said. "I could tell the minute I saw you two rollin' 'round. Any more ready an' he'd best get you to a room. After the church nuptials, of course."

"Course," Caleb said. "So, Lily? Will you marry me?"

Her head rapidly bobbed. "Yes. Soon as possible." She latched onto him and kissed him again.

Caleb had most definitely come home.

"Caleb?" Isaac raced to him and grabbed hold. Seconds later, Horace and Lucas added their arms.

"Pa!" Noah toddled over as fast as his little legs could manage and joined them.

"Did he say, Pa?" Isaac asked.

Horace looked from Caleb to Noah, then his eyes widened. "Yep. He did. Makes sense now how all this happened."

"What?" Isaac couldn't look more confused.

"Caleb an' Lily." Horace threw up his hands. "Isaac, Noah's their baby."

"Oh." Isaac peered up at Caleb. "That mean you're gonna live here now?"

"Yep."

"What 'bout her?" He pointed behind Caleb.

"Uh-huh. Her, too. She's my ma." He shifted his eyes to Mr. Larsen, who hadn't taken *his* eyes off her.

"Gamma," Noah said.

Lily lifted him. "Mrs. Quincy's gonna have more to talk 'bout."

Caleb chuckled and put his arm around Lily. "I'd like to meet Mrs. Quincy face to face. Last time I was anywhere close to her, I was behind a curtain. Course, I could wear your old dress an' pretend to be Callie."

"That wouldn't work. I told her Callie died. You'll hafta wear pants, but I prefer you that way."

He bent to give her another kiss, not caring who was watching. After all, they were all family now.

She puckered her lips, but Caleb stopped and sniffed. "Is sumthin' burnin'?"

Lily's eyes popped wide. "Oh, my!" She raced into the kitchen. "I forgot to flip the chicken."

Caleb gazed heavenward, shook his head, and grinned.

Chapter 36

Lily grasped tightly onto her pa's arm. "I wish I woulda had time to invite Mrs. Gottlieb, an' Archibald, an' the Jacobsons, an' all my other friends."

"The most important folks is here." Her pa kissed her cheek. "Them others are here in spirit. Just like your ma. I know they'll all be happy for you."

He guided her down the center aisle of the small church. Though not dressed in white, Lily wore the fancy blue gown she'd gotten from Aunt Helen. The beautiful collar tatted by Arabelle made it special.

All that truly mattered was Caleb, who stood at the front of the church, waiting for her.

The preacher had been a little befuddled when she and Caleb asked him to marry them, but Lily knew Brother Davis had heard all the gossip.

Some folks claimed Lily had been working as a harlot on a steamboat in St. Louis. Others said she was living with a man and his family in Asheville as his mistress.

Hateful gossip never did anyone any good.

Caleb and Lily had told Brother Davis the truth and he readily agreed to perform the ceremony.

They'd invited the congregation, but only a handful attended. Mrs. Quincy sat with her grandsons on the back pew. She'd likely come so she could be the first to tell stories. Yet, Lily decided to give her the benefit of the doubt. Maybe she had a heart and felt poorly for spreading ugly rumors.

Lily's pa placed her hand in Caleb's, then he took the seat next to Mrs. Henry and Avery.

Lily glanced at Violet, who of course was sitting in the front row with Gideon and his folks. Lily's brothers sat beside them, Lucas holding Noah on his lap.

Violet beamed. She shifted her eyes toward their pa and Mrs. Henry. Lily's sister had become a matchmaker.

Honestly, Lily saw it as the perfect fit. Her pa was a good man and Mrs. Henry a fine woman. And as Violet had always said, no one should be alone.

Lily put her full attention on the man she loved. He looked so handsome in his gray suit.

They'd had their share of kisses since his arrival, but she longed to be closer. Even so, she abided by her pa's wishes. That closeness would come later tonight.

"Caleb Henry," the preacher said. "Do you take Lily Larsen to be your wife? To have and to hold from this day forward. For better, for worse, for richer, for poorer, in sickness an' in health, to love, an' to cherish, till death do you part?"

Caleb shifted toward her and stroked her cheek. "I do."

Lily felt the dreaded tears again.

The preacher repeated the same words for her and of course she said, "I do."

"Please face me," Brother Davis said.

Caleb tightened his hold on Lily's hand and they turned toward the preacher.

"The two of you have come before God an' these witnesses and have shared your vows." He paused and gazed out at the congregation. "No two love stories are ever alike. When I met this fine couple, I had heard some ugly things bein' said 'bout them. Perhaps there are some of you here who are hangin' onto the lies that were told. I pray that as people of God, we can set those things aside an' learn how to lift each other up, rather than tear one another down.

"Christ taught us forgiveness. He sacrificed Himself so that we can live forever. He set an example for all of us to follow. I ask that you embrace this young couple an' their children in Christian love an' welcome them openly to our church family."

Lily squeezed Caleb's hand.

"An' now . . ." Brother Davis stood tall and smiled. "I pronounce you husband an' wife. You may kiss your bride."

Caleb drew Lily into his arms and kissed her—as the preacher said—before God and all their witnesses.

"Ma!" Noah jumped from Lucas's lap and put himself between Lily and Caleb.

"Pa!" Avery followed suit.

They each picked up a child and paraded with them down the aisle.

Lily's heart danced. All her hopes, prayers, and wishes had been answered. Yes, they'd have to work hard to build a home, raise the children, and keep the crops thriving, but she wouldn't be doing it alone. Her best friend, lover, and husband would be by her side. Till death parted them.

* * *

Caleb brightened the lamp on the stand next to the bed.

"Why'd you do that?" Lily rested her head on the pillow, looking so beautiful he could scarcely breathe.

"So I can see you." He laid down beside her and ran a single finger around her face.

He appreciated that Gideon and Violet had loaned them the little cabin for the night. Violet had called it a weaner house. A term he'd not heard before, but he understood its meaning.

He and Gideon had cabins to build, but for tonight, he didn't want to think of anything but Lily. The children were with their grandparents and he and Lily might not get this opportunity again for a great while.

She threaded her fingers into his hair. "I've always loved your thick hair." She smiled and unfastened the top buttons on his shirt. "*This* hair, too." Her fingers glided in slow circles over his chest.

"What 'bout my whiskers?"

Her head drew back. "You don't have any."

"I know. I shaved cuz I know you prefer it that way." He grinned and gave her a quick peck. "Sometimes, I noticed you talk real proper like, then other times you sound like my old Lily."

"Which way do you prefer?"

"Any way I can get you." He sat up and removed his shirt. "I recall a time when you said you wanted to do this every night."

"Do what?" She coyly tilted her head, then let out a tiny giggle. "Are you tryin' to embarrass me?"

"The Lily Larsen I know don't get embarrassed." He undid his trousers, then tossed them on the floor. "If I'm not mistaken, you ain't wearin' nothin' under them blankets. Am I right?"

She worked her lower lip and nodded.

Without a bit of hesitation, he stripped bare and got beneath the quilts.

Lily cuddled into him and buried her face in his neck. "I love you more than ever, Caleb Henry."

"I reckon that means you've forgiven me for bein' a fool."

She lifted her head and moved her face within inches of his. "It wasn't foolish to marry Rebecca. I always understood."

"An' it don't bother you knowin' that she an' I—"

"Hush." She pressed her hand to his mouth. "It's you an' me now. Forever. Just love me. Please?"

He closed his eyes and kissed her with passion that had been bottled up inside him for years. He'd imagined this moment for a long time, but never thought he'd actually be blessed with it.

They joined differently than they had when they were younger and inexperienced. This held a different kind of fire.

They lit up the night with an eternal flame that would last forever.

Epilogue

"It's comin!" Lucas yelled. His frantic green eyes told Lily all she needed to know.

"Go in the field an' tell Pa an' Caleb. I'll get the wagon ready."

Lucas raced out the door.

Lily's heart pattered harder. She prayed the delivery would have no complications.

"Boys!" she yelled up into the loft. "C'mon. Violet's havin' her baby!"

Thundering footsteps came down, followed by a very slow Noah, who took each stair one by one.

Lily picked Avery up from the floor. She'd been singing to Moo Cow. "C'mon sweetheart. We gotta go see the new baby."

"Baby cow?"

"No. Baby person."

She shuffled them out the door.

Horace hitched the horses to the wagon and everyone climbed inside. "Isaac. You help Horace keep an eye on the little ones."

They each wrapped an arm around the toddlers.

The heat of the July day didn't help. Once they'd gathered the men and reached the Myers' cabin, everyone was covered in sweat.

Mrs. Henry had been with Violet since the previous night. She'd had experience as a midwife. Caleb had told Lily that his ma had been with Rebecca when she'd delivered Avery. And in the short time Mrs. Henry had been in the cove, they'd all grown fond of her. Violet had specifically asked her to deliver her child.

Gideon and his pa met them all on the front stoop.

Gideon looked fit to be tied. "It's a girl!" He stumbled toward Caleb, who caught him and helped him steady himself on his crutch.

Lily cried happy tears. "How's Violet?"

"Strong an' feisty." Gideon grinned, then panted several breaths and sobered. "Hurtin' a mite, too, but Mrs. Henry said she did well. Said she was meant to have babies. Reckon that means we'll have more."

"Have you named her?" Caleb asked.

"Yep. Ivy Rose."

Lily's pa wiped his eyes. "Rose would be proud."

"I like it," Lily said. "Can I see her?"

Gideon patted his face with his shirtsleeve. "Ma an' Mrs. Henry is cleanin' up little Ivy, but Violet's been askin' for you."

"Good. I'm dyin' to see her." The excitement and joy of the situation had Lily chompin' at the bit. She grabbed onto Caleb. "Mind waitin' here with the children so I can have a minute with my sister?"

"Take as long as you need." He kissed her, then rounded up the kids.

"Thank you!" She wasted no time, flew into the house, and went to Violet's side. "You all right?" She stroked her sister's damp head.

"I am now. Have you seen my baby?"

"Not yet. The gramma's are hoggin' her, but I'll get my chance." Lily laughed and made herself comfortable on the edge of the bed.

Violet grabbed her hand. "Ivy's so beautiful, Lily. She has Gideon's eyes an' my nose."

"I like the name you chose. Maybe for my next baby I should choose a plant instead of a flower." She grinned. "Sumthin' like Fern."

"Oh. That's a good one. We might as well start a new family tradition."

Lily pulled her hand to herself and placed it on her stomach. "I might be keepin' it goin' sooner rather than later."

"You think you're with child?" Violet whispered.

"I do."

"Have you told Caleb?"

"Not yet, but I will." Lily and Caleb had somehow managed to work things out so they frequently had quiet time alone together. They'd even snuck off to the old hollowed out hillside on one occasion. It was no wonder she'd already conceived.

Violet beamed. "We're gonna have amazin' family celebrations." She turned her head toward the kitchen. "Ma? Is Ivy all clean?"

Mrs. Myers walked over with a blanketed bundle in her arms. "She's the most precious thing I ever seen." She laid her in Violet's arms.

Lily pulled back the covering and peered at Ivy's tiny face. Absolutely perfect features.

Mrs. Henry smiled down at them. "I'm gonna go out an' let Buck know all's well in here. I'm sure he's been frettin' over Violet."

"You go on, Ma," Lily said.

"I'm goin' with her," Mrs. Myers said. "Give you more alone time."

Lily gestured to the baby. "Can I hold her?"

"Course." Violet eased her into Lily's arms.

"Violet? Do you still wish you'd left the cove? You always said you wanted to."

"No." Violet tenderly ran her fingers across the top of Ivy's head. "This is my home. I was a silly young girl who didn't know what was important. Now I do."

Lily nodded. "I'm glad. I want you close forever." She swayed with Ivy, then closed her eyes and breathed in the scent of her newborn niece.

Life in the cove *had* changed since the war.

It had finally become far better.

Acknowledgments

It's incredibly bittersweet coming to the end of this series. And perhaps my heart is telling me that I'm not yet finished with stories from the cove. I couldn't bring myself to type the words, THE END.

We'll see . . .

Thank you so much for traveling to the Smoky Mountains with me and sharing Lily and Caleb's journey.

I enjoyed adding Asheville as a location in this book. And just as I encouraged you to visit Cades Cove, I highly suggest you make a stop in Asheville, North Carolina. The Biltmore Estate alone is a great reason to go there. It's breathtaking. As a lover of history, I enjoy visiting places that have retained their historical atmosphere and keep their buildings much as they were when they were constructed. You will definitely find yourself walking back in time when you tour the Biltmore. Though it wasn't part of this story—since it was built years after the time period *Murmurs* was set—it captures the beauty and magnificence of the area, and I just had to mention it. :)

I owe a great deal of gratitude to a very special lady who I consulted while writing this book. I met Duanne Puckett when I first moved to Shelbyville, Kentucky. Duanne is a journalist who interviewed me for an article she wrote for Shelby County Life magazine. I immediately liked her, but more than that, I was impressed by her incredibly bright attitude and positive outlook on life.

At the age of sixteen, Duanne was paralyzed from the neck down, when a drunk driver hit the car she was riding in with several friends. She never let the accident stop her from living a full and productive life. Duanne graciously shared her experience with me and gave me great insight into what it would be like for Arabelle to cope with day-to-day living.

Thank you, Duanne, for inspiring me and helping me bring Arabelle to life.

I'd also like to thank Cindy Brannam. My editor and my rock. She keeps me on task and helps polish my stories to a shine. Her encouragement is priceless. Thank you also to the rest of my team, Rae Monet, Jesse Gordon, and Karen Duvall.

I had two Beta readers for this project: Diane Gardner and Charli Heyer. They're both fast and efficient readers, and I appreciate that they took the time to go through my manuscript and share their honest opinions. Thank you!

For all you readers who sent me emails, Facebook messages, and notes through my website, thank you for being so excited and eager to read this book! I'd love to hear from you and know your thoughts on whether or not you'd like to see this series continue. Whose story would you like me to tell? Please send your thoughts to my direct email: hardtjeanne@gmail.com

I plan to keep the books coming. In 2018, I'll be releasing a medieval novel. A love story called *Island in the Forest*. I'll also be working on a new saga set in the Rocky Mountains, based on a true story from one of my dear friends. Stories keep running through my mind, and as long as I can type, I'll keep writing.

God Bless!

Jeanne

Books by Jeanne Hardt

The River Romance Series:
Marked
Tainted
Forgotten

From the Ashes of Atlanta

A Golden Life

The Southern Secrets Saga:
Deceptions
Consequences
Desires
Incivilities
Revelations
Misconceptions
Redemption

He's in My Dreams

The Smoky Mountain Secrets Saga:
Whispers from the Cove
Hushed into Silence
Murmurs in the Mountains

For more information about Jeanne's books,
check out the links below:

www.facebook.com/JEANNEHARDTAUTHOR
www.jeannehardt.com
www.amazon.com/author/jeannehardt
www.goodreads.com/jeannehardt

Made in the USA
Middletown, DE
28 December 2018